TABLE OF CONTENTS

Forward

This is the part of the book, where every self-help author, and every self-proclaimed guru, will have dozens of blurbs and words of praise, from clients, experts, and trusted celebrities, endorsing their brand.

I want to be totally honest with you.

Of the millions and billions of smokers, overweight people, sad people, abused people, only the tiniest fraction of a fraction, will ever seek help from me, or any other hypnotist.

Even if all the hypnotists in the world helped their clients 100% of the time, there are still not enough hypnotists to solve everyone's problems.

And if I can be even more honest than all the other hypnotists out there, I will add that many of my clients do not find the behavior changes they are looking for. Some are too distracted with worries, fears, or grief. Others have allowed their own opinion of themselves to erode to something so small, they simply can't find it.

Most hypnotists will describe hypnosis in terms of science, using psychology, neurological terms like theta brainwaves. I prefer to

Alex the Hypnotist has written a must read primer for anyone trapped in a bad habit. If you are struggling with addiction, weight loss, or smoking, you need to read this book, and learn from one of the best." - Mary Lou Rodriguez, CHT, Life Guidance Hypnosis, Beaverton, Oregon

This book is going to change your life: Learn how to break any bad habit, stop intrusive thoughts, procrastination, negative self talk, self sabotage, and more. Included are hypnosis scripts to hypnotize anyone easily.

Are you struggling with a bad habit?

Do you want to quit smoking, or lose weight, easily, and without cravings?

Are you tired of feeling afraid, sad, angry or hopeless?

Hypnosis is the answer.

The magic power of hypnosis has been healing people since before recorded history. Recent scientific advancements have expanded the potential of what hypnosis is capable of. With this book you can learn how to hypnotize anyone, and help them break unwanted habits, lose weight, stop smoking, and feel good about themselves.

In this book, you'll learn:

- How to break any bad habit
- How to stop intrusive thoughts and "junkie thinking"
- Discover why we procrastinate, and how to stop it
- Recognize self sabotage and stop it in its tracks
- Learn powerful hypnotic inductions you can use to hypnotize anyone
- Unleash your true potential, by unlocking the power of your subconscious

This book is going to change your life in a way you can't even imagine. Discover the awesome magic inside yourself, the power to stop bad habits, negative thinking, addictions, and self sabotage.

About the Author

Alex the Hypnotist has hypnotized hundreds of people all over the world, on every continent, and every English speaking country. Alex uses online video calling by Skype and Messenger to hypnotize clients internationally, helping them break bad habits, stop feeling sad, lose weight, and reach for the stars.

Since he was a young boy, Alex has dreamed of helping people solve life's biggest problems. After years of research and study, Alex began practicing hypnosis professionally, and his efforts have dramatically improved the lives of countless people, helping them feel better, live healthier, and smile more.

Alex lives in a small town in Michigan, with his lovely wife and two dogs that mean the world to him.

describe hypnosis as a form of magic.

Some people believe in their own personal magic. They believe hypnosis can change the way they think and feel and behave. For these lucky people, hypnosis truly is magical.

For the others, I feel sad for them.

When I see a depressed woman, lost in grief and self hatred, talking about suicide, and I tell her that I believe she is under a "curse", that she was labeled, "Depression" or "PTSD" or "Generalized Anxiety Disorder," by a powerful coven, the American Psychiatric Association, and she needs to believe that there is truly nothing wrong with her, she will resist my suggestion, because it means she was fooled, tricked, and that she suffered for so many years when she really didn't have to.

She believes she is mentally sick. If hypnosis can't help her, I don't know what can. All I know is, hypnosis has a better track record of healing people, than pharmacy psych meds.

Hypnosis is an incredibly personal process. I have not figured out how to mass-produce and mass-market the tools of hypnosis effectively. Most hypnotists sell books, and MP3 recordings, but without the personal touch and influence of a hypnotist, these products do not produce lasting results. Yes, I frequently give my clients MP3 recordings, that they play as they sleep at night. But I don't pretend like that is the cure. At best, the recordings improve their chances of success.

People need a personal touch. They need to meet me, and learn to trust me. I hold them accountable when they get lazy, I calm them when they get scared, I inspire them when they feel like giving up. This can't be done with an MP3 recording, or a book.

I have hypnotized over 1,000 people online, by skype and Messenger video calling. I offer low cost and even free hypnosis to people on Facebook and Reddit. I love to help people, and I love the practice. People are so grateful, they give me donations, and good reviews.

Not all of my clients reach their goals. Are you surprised at my honesty? All the other gurus tell you about how great they are, but they never discuss the clients who fail. I want to be honest with you.

Most people who call me never make it to the hypnosis session! Change is scary. Giving up is easy.

We are all guilty of self sabotage. That means we know what we ought to be doing, to live the kind of life we truly want. But this means stepping out of our comfort zone, and sadly we find that to be difficult, scary.

The truth is, about 20% of my clients are easy to hypnotize. They come in, I do my magic, and they leave, totally ready for success in reaching their goal.

Then there is the other end of the spectrum. Roughly 20% of my clients are too stressed, too depressed, too mistrusting of hypnosis, or strangers in general, to relax enough for hypnosis. In these situations, I rely on my life coaching skills.

You are probably somewhere in between. Hypnosis will definitely help you, but for the best results, you will need multiple sessions, and you need a clearly defined plan of action, to help you reach your goal.

I help who I can. Like any professional, I practice constantly, adding new techniques to my toolbox. I don't like to brag about my success, but when I sit and think of all the people I've helped to quit smoking, lose weight, reduce chronic pain, deal with depression, phobias, and sexual problems, I can't help but smile. I am making a huge difference in so many people's lives, and that makes me feel wonderful inside.

I want to help you too. As the reader of this book, you may already be my client. I am honored to be your guide on this magical journey, as I help you solve your life's biggest problems.

I conduct every session with an attitude of caring friendship. I strive to give each client the best advice, at the perfect moment. If you try to give up, I will help you find fresh motivation. If you stumble, I will pick you up, and set you back on the path. I will guide you towards a happier, healthier YOU.

My fees are reasonable, and whenever I see someone struggling financially, I waive my fee. I believe in Karma, and I feel a deep satisfaction, when I help someone stop their destructive behavior.

I hope you enjoy this book, and if you are interested in sharing your story with me, I would love to hear it. My email is funwithhypnosis@gmail.com

Namaste,

Alex the Hypnotist

Acknowledgments

I want to thank Rhonda Byrne, author of "The Secret". This book changed my life, and if you haven't read it, you really need to stop what you're doing, right now, and read it. When I first read it, I felt so inspired, I wanted to stop strangers on the street, to share this book with them. Sadly, I discovered that the book's wisdom really is a secret, and virtually invisible, to the vast majority of people who need it the most.

Tony Robbins is a modern day healer and an inspiration to me. Did you know he started as a hypnotist?

Stephen Covey, Norman Vincent Peale, and Joseph Campbell are among the Visionaries who left a lasting impression on me. If you have not read their books you really should.

My favorite hypnotists include Igor Ledochowski, Anthony Jacquin, Milton Erickson, Gerald Kein, Don Spencer, and my favorite, Cal Banyan.

I thank you all for sharing your wisdom and experience with me.

Hypnosis, Yoga, and Meditation

The more I study and practice hypnosis, yoga, and meditation (HYM), the more I see that they are like fingers on the same hand. They seem different, but they are deeply connected.

For most of my clients, hypnosis is a one-time thing. But meditation is a daily thing, and yoga can be too, so the benefits are huge, including reduced stress, increased positivity, better sleep, and clearer thinking.

If you are trying to break a bad habit, your enemy is stress and boredom. Meditation and yoga can make you feel happy, all by yourself, just observing the rhythm of your own breath, stretching your muscles to release built-up tension. Meditation and yoga will give you what smoking and overeating only promise— stress reduction and a feeling of genuine satisfaction.

This book is about hypnosis, and breaking bad habits, so I won't go into details about meditation and yoga. Let me just say that I recommend meditation more than anything else, to my clients.

This book is about habits. Please understand, that if you try meditation for an hour or two, you won't get much. You need to make it a daily ritual, no matter how busy you are. In fact, the more busy you are, the more you need to do daily meditation.

I do yoga once a week, but many clients do yoga daily. You can attend a local class, which I prefer, or you can watch videos on YouTube, like "Yoga by Adriene."

Meditation makes the modern (human) parts of the brain stronger, and the animal impulses weaker. Over time, you will develop the ability to ignore intrusive thoughts, negative feelings, and most of all, you won't feel compelled to surrender to an intense feeling, like the junkie impulse to smoke a cigarette.

Your greatest chance for successfully breaking your bad habit, is to incorporate relaxation techniques like meditation and yoga, into your daily routine. When you experience high levels of stress, or powerful negative emotions, you risk relapse. Yoga and meditation will lower your stress, and reduce the intensity of any negative emotions, so you can confidently change your behavior.

I Am What I Believe I Am

Our minds are maleable, plastic, and can be formed into a shape of our choosing....

The first thing we must do, to live a happy life, is tame our own mind.

Intrusive thoughts, self sabotage, destructive habits, these dangerous thought patterns are habits, and we can break these bad thought patterns, and replace them with better ones.

Meditation is the answer. By practicing mindfulness, we can develop a habit, of quick and complete mental relaxation, anytime. We just decide to focus on our breathing, and we slip into a state of pleasant mental calm. Because we practice daily, frequently, the habit becomes permanent. Relaxation quiets the storm of unwelcome and intrusive thoughts.

It is impossible to be happy, with an untamed mind. Sure, you can experience moments of pleasure, small events where you feel satisfied, but they cannot last. And the reason is because an intrusive thought can interfere with your happiness, and ruin it.

Let's say you get a raise at work. You are so happy! But here come the stupid thoughts... "Maybe my boss gave me a raise, because he's going to increase my workload?" "Should I tell my wife about my raise? She'll just waste the money on more shoes for herself." "The raise was rather small, don't I deserve a bigger one?"

What should have been a cause for celebration has been ruined by intrusive thoughts.

By practicing meditation, we learn to stop the constant chatter and interference of all thoughts. We focus on our breathing, giving all our energy and attention to the feeling of the air as it passes in and out of the lungs, the nose, the mouth. If we get distracted by a stray thought, we just gently redirect our mind to our breathing.

Trust me, it gets easier, the more you practice. At first, 5 minutes of mindful meditation is a challenge, but with practice, you will extend that time more and more, and the deeper you go the better you will feel.

The reason most of us are trapped in a bad habit is....STRESS.

We consciously want to stop the habit, but when we feel stressed, our mind defaults to the reptilian brain, a habit center, and this part of the brain selects a method to reduce the stress, by asking itself, "How did we treat this stress the last time?"

If we normally treat stress with a cigarette, or some fast food, then that's what we will reach for in times of stress. It's a coping mechanism, a habit that temporarily distracts us from the stress, but usually doesn't eliminate it.

If the stress reliever really worked, you would call it a good habit, not a bad one.

No, eating donuts is not a great way to deal with our feelings, following an argument with our spouse. But it makes us feel better temporarily. It is a bad habit, because the bad feelings soon return, forcing us to reach for yet another snack or cigarette.

We do not have to live at the mercy of an untamed mind.

The way we are, right now, is the consequence of the way we have thought and acted, up to now.

Everything about us is habitual. The more we entertain a thought, or a particular type of thought, the more our minds are prone, to generate thoughts of that nature.

Intrusive Thoughts

The way to deal with any thought that is dangerous or just plain stupid, is to treat it as if it was spam. For example, cigarette smoking is dangerous because of cancer and heart attacks and it also happens to be very stupid.

So what usually happens for a new non smoker, is he will feel great about his decision to quit smoking. But he has a constant pestering self-talk taking place. And this is all his addiction talking. I call it "Junkie Thinking." The addiction says things like, "Why don't you smoke a cigarette?" or, "You'll never get through this day unless you smoke a cigarette."

Does that sound familiar?

The mistake that most of us make is we try to placate and satisfy the pleas of the addiction, by explaining that smoking is bad, and we have promised ourselves we were going to quit, Etc and so forth. It is easy to forget that we are speaking with a deadly addiction. And this addiction is going to kill us if we continue to talk to it and try to reason with it.

But the more mental and emotional energy we give to cigarettes, the more powerful the thought becomes. Did you ever notice how the urge to smoke can almost force you to do shameful things, like begging, or even stealing a cigarette?

The solution is, to not think about smoking at all. When the thought comes up, we don't feel love, hate, anger, annoyance...we feel nothing at all. We label the thought SPAM, because we already decided to quit, and the subject is not open for discussion.

Nicotine is like a pushy salesman, knocking on your door. If you open the door, you will have to listen to his pitch, and you may end up buying something you don't really want. The best thing to do is not answer the door, and wait till he gives up and goes away.

Let some time pass, and I promise you, the thought, robbed of all emotional energy and attention, will shrivel up and disappear.

In order for the smoker to become a non-smoker, she has to stop communicating with the voice of her addiction. Any thoughts about cigarettes or smoking should be treated as if they were spam.

Spam is any thought that is dangerous or stupid, or that has already been decided upon. In life we cannot constantly question our decisions. Many times our decisions are so important we must make the right decision every time. This is one of those times.

Imagine if a judge let any criminal appeal his conviction, as many times as he liked, for any reason, or no reason at all! The court would lose all control. When a judge makes a judgement, it is final, and YOUR decisions should be final and absolute, just like a judge's.

False Alarms, Unimportant, Addiction, & Spam

So many of our thoughts are junk! Be honest with yourself. Examine your thoughts, and you will see that most of them do not serve you.

If you get a thought that says, "Did you remember to lock the front door?", you might consider this to be important. But what if this thought keeps coming at you, a dozen times a day? What if it makes you doubt your own memory, and wastes so much of your time, checking the door like a fool, only to find that it is actually locked every single time?

This thought is called a **FALSE ALARM**. Whenever this thought comes up, you should simply label it **FALSE ALARM**, and disregard it. Don't give it any attention at all, it is irrelevant, junk mail, it's like a neighbor's car, whose alarm is too sensitive, and his horn is blaring at all hours. Yes, it's annoying, but it's best to disregard it. NEVER have a dialogue with this voice, it is the voice of Worry, and the more you discuss locking doors, the more energy you give it, and the more frequently and powerfully the thought will return.

A **FALSE ALARM**, like any other junk thought, should be treated like spam. You label it, and forget about it. You never debate or discuss the thought, because it's attached to the feeling of Worry, and that's a negative emotion. You will never satisfy Worry with logical discussion. An internal dialogue, or self talk, gives a **FALSE ALARM** more power, so we simply label the thought, then disregard it.

Let's say you got in an argument with a coworker, and feelings got hurt. Your boss hears about it, and he asks you both to apologize and drop the matter. You apologize, and you want to forget the whole thing, but your mind just won't let it go. Over and over, you have thoughts about punching the coworker, or scratching his car. You tell yourself to stop thinking about revenge, but the thoughts just get stronger and more frequent.

This thought is what we call a sticky thought. Because hurt feelings are so powerful, this thought has its own energy source. The only way to stop this thought, is to label it **UNIMPORTANT**.

You have already decided to accept your coworker's apology, but your pride was hurt, and you keep thinking about revenge. Your decision is final and absolute, not to be debated or discussed.

When this thought returns, simply label it **UNIMPORTANT**, and think of something else, or nothing at all. Let some time pass, and as you continue to think of this thought as **UNIMPORTANT**, it will soon stop bothering you.

You feed a thought, by mentally discussing it, arguing with it, compromising, and giving it more importance than it deserves. Your brain is a very simple machine. If you feed a thought with emotions like sadness, fear, anger, or worry, the thought becomes stronger, and returns to mind frequently.

In a very short time, you can feed a negative thought so much, that it can become very strong indeed. It's as if a bully moved into your head, and started pushing you around, telling you to do things that are dangerous. Soon, a thought can grow so big, that you feel powerless to resist. Like a helpless puppet, the thought commands you to do things you really don't want to do.

We call this **ADDICTION**. You have let a dangerous habit spin out of control, and now you are afraid you might be addicted. This fear is actually feeding the thought, making it very powerful. You wonder if you can ever break free of this mental bully.

We stop this thought like any other negative or unwanted thought. For example, a smoker feels satisfied when he smokes, but over time, he regrets the side effects, and tries to quit. He fails. Now he's scared he might never break free from cigarettes. That fear feeds the thought, making the habit even stronger.

Thoughts are just thoughts. You can control your mind, but it will take effort and practice. If you are battling your **ADDIC-TION**, using will power, you will lose. The correct way to break the habit is, label any thought about smoking as **ADDICTION**. Then treat it the same way you treat an unimportant thought or a false alarm thought. You just ignore it. Never discuss the thought in your mind, and have zero feelings about the thought. You don't feel like smoking...you aren't afraid of smoking....you aren't avoiding cigarettes...you simply don't think about them at all.
You label the thought of smoking as **ADDICTION**, and you disregard it, ignore it, pretend it doesn't matter, because it really doesn't matter.

Now, if you are having trouble with any of these steps, it's because you haven't calmed your mind enough, by practicing meditation. Meditation lets you clear your mind from all random thoughts. Meditation is vital to controlling and eliminating negative thoughts and emotions.

Trust the process. Let time pass. I promise you, thoughts are just thoughts, they must be fed, by you, in order to exist in your mind. Stop feeding them with your attention, and they will dry up and disappear. If you are struggling with this process, you need to practice your meditation.

When an unwanted thought hits you by surprise, and you are struggling to gain control, it helps to just close your eyes, focus on your breathing, and let your mind relax. Soon, after some deep breathing and gentle rest, you will remember to lable the thought "unimportant", and just let your mind float to some other topic, or no topic at all.

The Story of Rat Park

When a lab rat was left <u>alone</u> in a cage, he had 2 bowls of water.

One was clean, the other laced with morphine. Which bowl would the rats drink from?

All the rats tested like this became addicted to morphine and died from overdose.

However, when the rats were placed in a cage <u>with other rats</u>, and offered cheese, sex, friends, colored balls and tunnels, and also the 2 bowls of water, 1 clean and 1 laced with morphine, NONE of the rats became addicted.

What can we, as hypnotists, learn from this?

- The rat (and the client), needs meaningful social activities.
- Boredom is bad for rats (and clients)
- We should keep our clients actively involved in recovery, by presenting a specific plan of action, that isn't boring
- If a client is lonely, they have a greater risk of addiction

Anatomy of an Addiction

An addiction has 3 main parts:

- See food(trigger), eat food(behavior), feel full(reward)
- See cool kids smoking(trigger), smoke (behavior), feel cool(reward)
- Feel Sad(trigger), eat food(behavior), feel full(reward)

Our goal in hypnosis is to replace the old behavior (overeating, or smoking), with a healthier one (choosing an apple as a snack, or a Life-Saver instead of a cigarette).

We need to FEEL rewarded, when we choose the apple. Otherwise, a new healthy habit will not form. When the client is eating the apple, she should FEEL satisfied, and happy about her decision.

It's as simple as congratulating herself, and smiling privately. Remember, personal satisfaction feels very good, and we can easily remember to smile while eating the apple, or the Life-Saver candy.

If the client feels deprived, miserable, or stressed out, while eating the apple, the new habit won't take root.

Nature rewards animals, when they eat food, by giving them a feeling of satisfaction. They feel full, and gratified. Thus, eating became a habit, and all animals benefit, by eating often.

The same with sex. The urge to mate is rewarded with the orgasm, which is the satisfaction we get from mating. The orgasm, while very powerful indeed, only lasts long enough to breed and mate.

We can never stop a bad habit, because as long as there is a trigger, and a reward, there is the urge to do the behavior.

Instead, we REPLACE the habit, with a healthy action, and we replace the reward (a full belly, or reduction or stress, or the climax of sex), with a better reward (a personal inward smile, a happy feeling, a pat on the back, a few minutes of meditation).

None of this is quick and easy. Time must pass, for a habit to develop. Be patient. Expect and plan for relapse and setbacks. Clients screw up. When they do, they should just take a quick nap (this calms them down, and lets the mind reset). When they wake from the nap, they should redouble their efforts, and proceed with the habit replacement, as if no relapse occurred.

Why Meditation and Yoga is So Important

I promote yoga and meditation constantly to my clients, for many reasons.

First, I know that people often overeat, or smoke, or take drugs, as a way to deal with stress. Clients come to me, to break a destructive habit, and when I take away their imperfect method of dealing with stress, I need to replace it, with a better one.

Meditation and yoga are the most relaxing ways I know, to reduce stress, lower your blood pressure, clear your mind, and feel good about yourself.

Sadly, many of my clients never even try to meditate. But here's the sad fact- The ones that do try meditation, reach their goals faster, and they are also less likely to relapse.

The reason is simple.

Meditation actually makes you a better person! Over time, you become calmer, nicer, less grouchy. You learn how to dismiss intrusive thoughts with less effort, and just disregard them. You learn to avoid emotional traps of negativity. You are friendlier, more patient, and you smile more. You learn the value of restraint, when you feel a negative emotion inside, and this dramatically improves your behavior.

Before meditation, I used to feel uncomfortable in social situations. Now, I can actually enjoy these same activities, perfectly at ease.

On planet Earth, stressful situations, and unpleasant people, are everywhere. But by practicing daily meditation, I can prevent myself from feeling uncomfortable, and even if I do feel annoyed, I remind myself that this feeling will pass, and it does. Every single time.

If you don't know how to meditate, you should google 'Beginning

Meditation', and watch a YouTube video. It's so easy, you might doubt that it can be so powerful. Just give it a chance. Try it, for at least 5 minutes a day, for a month, and you will discover a new you, one that's calmer, happier, and more pleasant to be around.

Stress is a killer. And unfortunately, people are dying from stress everyday. People smoke, drink, use drugs, and do a hundred other dangerous things, just to relieve stress.

But all I have to do, when someone is rude or angry, and is close to pissing me off, is close my eyes, breathe deeply, and focus on my breathing. I empty my mind of all negative emotions, all distracting and destructive thoughts, and in just 5 minutes, I am calm, neutral, and ready to deal with the rude jerk, in a professional, non-confrontational way.

Meditation is a simple way to tell your body and mind, that everything is OK. We give ourselves permission to relax, and unplug.

When I used to be a loan officer, in California, I would stress so much! I couldn't sleep, I smoked, I drank too much, I got stress headaches, and upset stomach. I wish I knew about meditation and yoga back then!

To me, yoga is like meditation, but in a group. At first, I found it hard to relax in a room full of strangers. To be honest, I found it hard not to admire the beautiful women around me, in their yoga pants, doing poses like Downward Dog. But over time, my focus changed, and I don't see the women in a sexual way anymore. Every woman, old or young, large or petite, is like my yoga sister, a friend, and I never want to make any woman feel unconfortable. I am never a creep, I don't leer or stare. I just focus on my practice, and my mind is totally at peace. (Plus, my wife goes to yoga with me! We also go to the gym together, and I would never dishonor her, by staring or leering like a high school boy).

Yoga is like an active form of meditation, one that's guided by a teacher. When we ask our body to hold a pose, we gently insist on body/mind harmony, and contemplative stillness.

When I was first learning to meditate, the instruction was to simply pay attention to my breath, and when my mind wandered, to bring it back.

If you are struggling with meditation, or yoga, you can email me, and I will share some excellent instructional videos with you. Funwithhypnosis@gmail.com

Change Your Environment!

Changing your environment can dramatically improve your chances of breaking a bad habit.

If a heroin addict moves, from Los Angeles to Butte, Montana, he is much more likely to stay clean. In L.A., he knew where to get drugs, but in Montana, it's so much harder to find a dealer. Eventually, he will find one, but because it's not easy, he will spend a few days, or even weeks, sober, and that gives him a chance to stay sober on his own.

For most addicts, moving far away from his old drug hangouts is not an option. But most drug addicts need a residential treatment center anyway, in order to kick the habit. My advice is to choose a rehab center that's far away from your old neighborhood, as this will make it easier to ignore the 'junkie voice' in your head, begging for dope like a crying baby.

If you can't move far away, you should at least change your immediate environment. Take your phone, and delete or block all the numbers for drug associates and dealers. Tell your drug friends to stop calling or visiting you. Tell them you are quitting dope, and ask them to respect your decision. If they try to get you to use dope again, they are dangerous, selfish, and you should cut them out of your life completely. Even if your own brother, or mother, or wife, tries to sabotage your sobriety, you should avoid them.

Another way you can change your environment, without moving to another city, is to get rid of all the 'props' that support the idea of using. For example, a smoker must toss out all his ashtrays and lighters. An alcoholic must throw away his keychain bottle opener, and his T-shirts with beer logos.

Music is yet another way to change your environment. For me, music has a huge influence on my behavior. Certain genres, and certain songs, make me think of the bad habits I used to do, long ago, while I listened to that music. That's why I can't listen to System Of A Down, Slipknot, or Pink Floyd. Their songs have become triggers for me.

Instead, I listen to psybient music, calm, upbeat, positive, with very little vocals. This music makes it easy for me to think about meditation, kindness, and good living.

Helping Others

Why is helping others so important?

The answer is complicated, but I will try to explain it.

The biggest reason I ask my clients to help others, is because most habits are incredibly selfish ones. A man addicted to gambling will mortgage the family home, to feed the greed of the casino. A woman addicted to overeating doesn't care about the pain she is causing her husband and children, as they watch her slowly destroy her body. A mother who smokes cigarettes exposes her children to second-hand smoke, and she simply doesn't care enough about their health to take that poison outside.

When we are slaves to a bad habit, we learn to ignore the pain and complaints of the people around us. "They don't understand what I'm going through!" Wrong. Selfish behavior is nothing new or unique.

Here's the saddest part of being trapped in a selfish habit. Besides ruining the lives of their family and close friends, the subject is obviously unhappy too! They may pretend they are happy, stuffing their face with food, until they are too big to fit through the bathroom door, but inside they feel so rotten, so ugly, so guilty, so ashamed, and it's obvious to everyone they are not happy at all. Who can honestly claim to be happy, as they watch their lives, their bodies, their families, destroyed by a bad habit, and they are personally responsible for all the pain around them?

Logically, if the subject is unhappy, and her family is unhappy, then the habit serves no purpose at all. The only people who benefit from a bad habit are the greedy corporations, who sell obese people fatty foods, as the poor fat lady struggles to roll down the grocery aisle, on a mobility scooter, too fat to walk anymore, but still overeating, a diabetic, so many health problems, and the food corporations pretend this isn't happening everywhere.

The antidote for selfish behavior, is selfless behavior. Generosity, kindness, empathy, volunteering, cooperating, helping, these are the ways to break the cycle of selfish behavior permanently.

You must understand, that for the addict, there will NEVER be enough dope, or enough food, or enough anything. They will always want more, and that will always make them feel incomplete, dissatisfied, and empty.

The next big reason you should help others is this:

When you were behaving selfishly, you learned to ignore the pain you caused for others. Helping others repairs some of the damage you did. You may not be able 'make ammends' directly to the people you hurt; that is not always possible. But you can balance your Karma, by filling the lives of people around you with loving kindness, offsetting all the pain you caused previously.

The 3rd reason you should practice actively helping others, is to increase your own self respect. As an addict, compulsive gambler, overeater, or any other type of selfish person, your selfish behavior did great damage to your own self esteem. You feel guilty, weak, evil, ashamed, and afraid. By doing good deeds for others, you slowly feel better about yourself. When people compliment you on your good behavior, you feel less rotten. Soon, you will become "addicted" to helping others, and your own opinion of yourself will improve, because you are actually proud of your good deeds. You feel good, when you are doing good for others.

Ways to Practice Kindness

I think that for most of us, we really want to do good things for other people.

Sometimes, we "substitute" things for actual good deeds. A religious person might see a homeless person, and not give him any help, justifying her behavior by saying a quick prayer for the homeless. This is NOT kindness.

Other people will donate to the United Way, once a year, as if that makes it OK to ignore all the sick and dying people they see, all year long.

When I do good for someone, I feel good inside. I like the person I am, when I am acting friendly, thoughtful, and compassionately.

When I act kindly to someone, I don't do it for God to see me, and reward me.

I do it because I see myself doing good, and my opinion of myself improves.

My principles match my actions. Thus, there is no terrible conflict inside me. I am at peace.

"But Alex," you say, "What can I do to fix this screwed up world? Where do I even start? Can I even make a difference?"

I cannot help everyone. Sadly, there's not enough time or resources. So, I practice triage. I love dogs. They bring so much joy in my life, and they make me a better person. They give me love and make me very happy.

So, I do good things for dogs. I help shelter dogs find good homes. When I see a dog running around in the busy street, I stop my car and try to help. Dogs don't live very long, sadly. When my dog dies, and my heart has healed, I adopt another shelter dog, and share my love and home with my new best friend.

Now, I can't tell you what cause to take up. Maybe you're a cat person. That's great. Now go out and make the world a little better for cats.

Here's a clue-- If you suffered a lot of pain in life, you can use that pain, to reduce the pain of other people. For example, let's say you are the victim of sexual assault. Maybe you can volunteer to answer calls for crisis hotline, for victims of sexual assault, where they can connect to emergency services, like temporary housing, protection, and support groups.

In this way, you use the pain you went through, to prevent or reduce a similar pain for others.

This is how you heal. This is how you feel happy, all the time. You are making a difference.

Are you a former heroin addict? Why not start a recovery home, or a halfway house? You can make good money, and help addicts live better.

And the best part is, the pain you used to feel, is somehow easier to bear, because you are making a big difference to so many people.

You might be thinking, "I'm so busy! I'm broke too." There is a young girl in my town. She is handicapped. She paints the most beautiful "Kindness Rocks." These are small flat rocks, that she paints cheerful messages on. She writes things like, "You are Loved," "Smile and Be Happy," "You Rock," "Have Fun," "Don't Give Up." She may include a Peace Sign, or a red heart, or she might paint a flower or a sunset.

Then, she walks all over our small town, and places these Kindness Rocks in public places. Whenever I see one, I always smile and feel better.

If you don't know where to start, you can start with Kindness Rocks. If you are able to do something with more dramatic impact, go for it.

Your subconscious mind, your "conscience", will see your good deeds, and will change its opinion of you. Then something magic happens.   Your own subconscious will stop sabotaging you. Habits like smoking and drinking will lose any attraction. You will find a pure and permanent source for self satisfaction, the gratifying feeling of helping people, or animals, in a real and personal way.

Don't give money to United Way. You can do better. If there are homeless and hungry people in your city, don't give them your loose change. That's worthless. Why don't you open up a soup kitchen, or organize a canned food drive, or open a homeless shelter? Do something real, something significant, and watch how fast Karma comes in and lifts you up, blessing you for real, not just with a sense of personal value, but with prosperity of every type.

Here are some ways you can do good for the people in your neighborhood:

Kindness Rocks (www.thekindnessrocksproject.com)

Go to www.meetup.com, and start a group. Your group can be a support group, or an opportunity for people to make new friends. There are Meetup groups everywhere now, for almost every purpose. Check it out.

Go to www.7cups.com and volunteer to be a "listener." A Listener is a trained volunteer that offers emotional support to callers in crisis. You could save a life.

Save an Animals' Life. Help shelter dogs and cats find new homes with loving families. This feels so good, and is my favorite good deed.

Buy a stack of Post It Notes, and anonymously compliment and thank people. When you see a friendly face, or a generous co-worker, shopkeeper, or total stranger, just write a compliment on the Post It Note, and leave it where they will find it. I promise you will make them smile and feel wonderful.

Search YouTube and Facebook, for people practicing kindness and compassion, and give them a positive review or comment. You will feel wonderful, and the world will love it!

Sponsor a recovering addict or alcoholic in A.A. or N.A. You can help an addict get his life back, and that's the best feeling in the world.

Volunteer at a retirement home or hospital. The residents will be happy to see you. Friendship is magic.

Volunteer at the local school, as a tutor for math or reading. Children need help with their homework, and we all know how to read good enough to help a child with his homework.

Volunteer at a hospice. There is nothing scarier, or sadder, than a sick person dying all alone. You can stop this from happening, by just holding their hand, smiling, and sharing human contact. The experience will fill your heart with love.

Story of a Former Smoker

The first time I tried a cigarette and inhaled, I nearly choked to death.
And the taste of the smoke was disgusting.

But my need to fit in with my friends, and deal with stress and anxiety, made me go beyond my discomfort, and continue smoking.

I forced my mind and body to accept the smoke as normal.

And now I'm an addict.

But there's still hope.

You can quit smoking, with daily meditation and correct mental attitude.

Many years ago when I was in my early 20's I'd just started a new job.
I was sitting at a table in the staff restaurant with a group of people I didn't know.
They were all chatting together and I felt anxious and ill at ease.

Then someone offered me a cigarette.

Although I wasn't a regular smoker, I had smoked before.
So I took it and lit-up.
After taking a couple of puffs, I was transformed –
the nicotine coursing through my veins had made it to my brain within seconds.

I felt great – relaxed, confident and no anxiety.

Of course, I had to keep smoking to keep my brain flooded with nicotine.
And I realised that I'd have to become a regular smoker if I wanted the same effect.

But I knew this wasn't the answer.

Later, I learned how to use meditation to quit smoking or, I should say, <u>the smoking quit me.</u>

Because it wasn't an effort of will on my part – I just didn't want or need it any more.

I remember a friend of mine, Willis.

He would regularly smoke 60 cigarettes a day.
But he gave up smoking in a split-second, after a startling realisation.

He'd drive to various meetings and would smoke in the car.
At the start of the week he'd fill the car glove-box with packets of cigarettes.
Whilst driving he'd smoke and, when the packet was empty, he'd crush it and throw it into the passenger foot-well.

Then, at the end of the day he'd throw away the crushed packets .

On one particular day, he removed the old packets and to his horror realised that he'd smoked one hundred cigarettes.

He was so disgusted with himself that he never smoked a single cigarette ever again.

But what's even more amazing is that he didn't experience any withdrawal symptoms.
And never even had the slightest desire to smoke again.

His feeling of disgust, shocked him into awareness.

If you want to quit smoking you must cultivate this awareness.

Because the effect of the nicotine is to make you less aware.

But regular meditation will make you more aware.

Then, with this awareness, you can respond differently.
If you've tried to quit smoking, you've probably used will-power to resist the craving.
But your will-power is not as strong as the craving.
Although you may start out strong, slowly but surely your will-power will begin to shrink.
And eventually your will, will have no power at all.

Because using will-power is like struggling when you've fallen into a swamp –the more you struggle, the deeper you sink.

And you'll use up all your energy until you've got none left and you'll give up and give in.

So don't use will-power to stop smoking, use awareness instead.

When you feel the urge to smoke don't fight it, watch it.

Become fully aware of the feeling in your body.
When you take out your cigarettes, become aware of the weight and texture of the packet.
As you remove the celophane wrapping, become aware of the sound it makes.
When you take out a cigarette become aware of the smell of the tobacco.
Then, be aware as you put the cigarette in your mouth, light it and take a puff.
And an amazing thing will happen.
You'll be able to taste the true flavor of the smoke – **and it will be disgusting.**
And be fully aware of that too.

Everytime you smoke, go through this process as it were the first time you've done it.

But you must also keep up your regular meditation.
Eventually you won't even feel the need to smoke any more.
The pull won't be there. The attraction won't be there.
You'll start to feel as if you can take it or leave it.
And one day you'll leave it for good.

Then you'll be free.

And you'll have quit smoking completely –
without struggling and without withdrawal symptoms.

Smoking & Overeating

Within each of us, there are several "selves". We all have a "protector part" of us, in charge of keeping us safe. We have a "pleasure-seeking part", constantly looking to feel good. We have a "horny part", lust, and so on.

But did you know that we all have a destructive part?

The destructive part is the one that may act suicidal. This part "punishes" us, with self-destructive behavior.

There is a "healthy part" too, but for a smoker, this part is not nearly as strong as the destructive part.

Here are 3 things to remember about smoking:

    ☐☐ Smoke is a deadly poison to your body.
    ☐☐ Your body keeps you alive.
    ☐☐ If you want to live, you must protect and care for your body.

Smokers and overeaters treat their body horribly.

A big reason people ignore their destructive behavior, is because everyone knows that a single cigarette won't kill you. Neither will a single donut.

Again, meditation is the answer.

We meditate to increase our conscious awareness of our bodies. The more mindful we are to all the sensations of our bodies, the more we will want to protect and love our fragile, vital bodies, from all dangerous things.

Meditation reduces our stress. We know that when stress is high, our animal brain will override our higher brain, and push us toward "pleasure-seeking" behavior.

I know a man, who quit smoking for several years. One night, he was driving with his small daughter, and he was in a terrible accident. The car flipped, over and over, and from the back seat, he could hear his daughter screaming and crying. He was injured, and unable to help her at all.

It would be safe to say, this man was experiencing high stress.

After rescue crews arrived and pulled the man and his daughter from the wreck, the first thing the man did, was ask onlookers for a cigarette!

One cigarette led to another, and this man smoked heavy, for the next several years.

This is why meditation is so important. This man returned to smoking when faced with a moment of high stress. But even after the car accident, when his life calmed down, he continued smoking.

Addiction is a way of avoiding or transforming intolerable experiences (or stress) into something more manageable.

Both nicotine and food are able to quickly make us feel better, when we feel bad or stressed.

But cigarettes and snacks do nothing but mask the stress temporarily. Much better, to feel the stress, let it pass, and let it motivate us toward improving our situation, as best we can.

The man in the car accident, had he been a daily student of meditation, would have been better able to disregard unhealthy thoughts like begging strangers for a smoke. He would have been more empathetic to his daughter's pain, than on his own selfish emotional discomfort. If he felt stressed, he could have taken a cleansing deep breath, cleared his mind, and focused on his best course of action.

If he had did that, he would be a nonsmoker today.

Using Meditation to Quit Smoking

I frequently recommend meditation to my clients, whether they want to quit smoking, lose weight, reduce stress, sleep better, feel more confident, or even lower their blood pressure.

Rather than quote university studies that show how meditation can help a person with the problems mentioned above, I invite you to simply Google meditation research, and see for yourself.

From my experience, I can honestly say, that clients who use meditation to quit smoking, are more successful than those who don't.

Meditation, like hypnosis, may seem weird to many Americans. In India and China, meditation is common and accepted as a great way to reduce stress, worry, greed, uncertainty, and more.

I'm an American, so when I meditate, I like to sit in a flat-backed chair. I like to stare out at the river that runs through my backyard. This scene is so tranquil, it helps me relax quickly.

There is no need to twist your legs into a pretzel shape, unless you want to. For many Americans, sitting Indian style is painful, and meditation should feel pleasant.

Meditation is so important, if you have been wondering about it, please do yourself a big favor, and just try it, for 5 minutes a day, for at least 2 weeks. I promise you, the benefits you experience will make you a believer.

How do you meditate?

1. Sit in a chair, back straight, hands resting in your lap.
2. Close your eyes.
3. Focus on your breathing. Notice the way the air moves in and out, touching your nose, expanding your chest. Notice how your breath is sometimes soft, shallow, faint, or deep, loud, rapid, or somewhere in between, or different altogether. Just notice, and observe.
4. Whenever your thoughts stray to something else, just go back to #3, Focus on your breathing....

Many "experts" will try to complicate meditation, with mantras, difficult poses, etc. You are free to try any new style you discover, and see what works for you best. But as a beginner, all you need is the 4 steps above. My personal practice is focus on my breathing, and nothing else.

There are 3 main ways meditation helps you become a nonsmoker:

☐☐ **Meditation reduces stress, which is a big trigger for smoking.** People smoke because it makes them feel better when they are stressed out or worried. These people know smoking is bad—Everyone knows this! But they enjoy that brief moment of relaxation, after they take that first puff of a cigarette. By the time they get to the end of the cigarette, however, that good feeling is already fading fast. Soon, they will need to smoke another cigarette to feel relaxed. The truth is, smoking just covers up the stress, temporarily, but meditation can remove the stress permanently, and isn't that so much better? Daily meditation will lower your stress levels over time, and teach you how to manage any stressful situation better. With less stress in your life, you will have less reason to reach for a smoke in the first place.

☐☐ **Meditation trains you to be aware of your smoking habits and cravings.** Mindfulness is a term we use, to describe a heightened awareness of our own thoughts, feelings, and impulses. Usually, a bad habit is a behavior that is "automatic", requiring very little thought or attention. When I was addicted to nicotine, I remember how I would struggle and fight the urge to smoke. Then, when I became distracted, tired, or stressed, my struggles took a back seat, and the addiction "possessed" me. The addiction made me get up, get into my car, drive to the gas station, and buy a pack of smokes, like I was a mindless zombie. All the while, my conscious desire to quit smoking, was watching my body light up yet another cigarette, and I felt so defeated, so help-less. Over time, I felt like quitting was becoming harder and harder, because of so many failed attempts. Mindful-ness meditation will train you to SEE this addictive cycle for what it truly is. Addiction is not a choice! You don't choose to smoke, you are being bullied into smoking, by an addiction. Meditation helps you see the truth of your own behavior. Meditation allows you to accept the urge to smoke, without acting on it. We ignore the thought, just like we ignore all distracting thoughts, when we meditate, and focus on our breathing. Thoughts no longer push us around. Impulses that are dangerous or stupid no longer compel us to do anything we don't really want to do. We are free.

☐☐ **Meditation improves your self-control.** MRI brain scans have proven that daily meditation can actually change the structure of your brain. One way it does this, is by in-creasing the neural connectivity between parts of the brain responsible for self-control. And the more self-control you have, the easier it will be for you, to ignore and deflect any urge to smoke.

The 3 Parts of a Habit

At the core of every habit, is a loop that consists of three parts: A cue, a routine and a reward.

The Cue

This can be anything that triggers the habit.

Cues could fall under the following categories:

- *A location* (I always order onion rings at a certain restaurant)
- *A Time of Day* (I like a cup of coffee every morning at 6 a.m.)
- *Other People* (When I hang out with Joe, I drink too much)
- *An Emotional State* (I eat when I feel bored)

The Cue is what tells the brain to go into "automatic" mode. It takes effort to resist the cue. We feel satisfied when we follow the cue.

The Routine is the behavior you want to change. Smoking is a routine. Another is overeating. A routine can also be a new behavior you are trying to reinforce and make permanent. You may be replacing sugary snacks with fresh fruit, and thus creating a new routine.

The Reward is the reason your brain has decided to remember and repeat this behavior in the future. There must have been some benefit, or good feeling, as a payoff, and this is what reinforced the habit, made it permanent. The reward is positive reinforcement for the desired behavior. The reward can be anything seen as positive, from a compliment, to social acceptance, to a satisfaction of a basic need, like sex or hunger.

Here is how we break a habit--

☐☐　　**Identify the Routine** (The behavior you want to change). In this example, let's say the Routine is smoking.

☐☐ **Experiment with Rewards**. Rewards can be complex, and subtle. Is the client smoking because his girlfriend smokes? Is it to cope with stress? Is it to seem cool? Try substituting candy or chewing gum for a cigarette. Try meditation for 5 minutes, instead of smoking. Eat an apple, take a walk, almost anything can be a good substitute for smoking, as long as it's healthy and feels good.

☐☐ **Isolate the Cue**. This is not always easy. You can answer the following questions, to gain insight in what is triggering the habit:

1. Where are you (when the craving or urge strikes)?
2. What time is it?
3. How do you feel right now?
4. Who else is with you?
5. What happened just before you felt the urge?

Let's say a smoker notices the urge to smoke whenever it's break time at work. The whistle blows, and he automatically walks outside to smoke, finishing right about when break is over. While he's smoking, he chats with a few of the other smokers, about weekend plans, the weather, the usual stuff.

We might suggest that this smoker go to the cafeteria instead, and snack on a banana or apple. While he's there, he should make friendly chat with the other coworkers, to satisfy his social needs. As long as he tries to relax and enjoy his cafeteria detour, this new routine will get stronger over time, while the habit of going outside to smoke will get weaker.

Guided Meditation & Sleep Hypnosis

Every time a client calls me, no matter what their problem is, I always ask them for their email, so I can send them an MP3 recording. This Sleep Hypnosis recording is to be played several nights in a row, for best results.

As the client sleeps, the hypnotic words of the recording, soak into his subconscious, making my job so much easier.

Each recording is custom designed for the clients' specific problem. If a client has an odd or unique problem, and a good recording can't be found on that topic, I send them what I feel will help them the most. For example, if the client is afraid of being abducted by aliens, I probably won't find a recording on that narrow subject. So instead, I will send him a recording about overcoming phobias.

These recordings have several benefits. First, they are practically free. It costs me nothing to send a digital copy to a client. Second, the internet is full of free or almost free hypnotherapy content, especially these types of audio recordings, made by literally every major hypnotist out there.

But most of all, when a client calls me, they feel alone, uncertain, and often helpless. When I send them this recording, I want them to feel like I deal with this problem everyday, and I have a plan to help.

Most clients will probably not listen to the MP3's. But for the ones that do, the reward is a much higher probability for success.

"Sorry, I didn't listen to it, I had such a busy week." Really? If a smoker claims he was too busy to listen to it, I may remind him that he found the time to smoke 60 cigarettes yesterday, but no time to listen to the recording? It's supposed to be played at night, as they sleep, so how is it they don't have the time? It's a lousy excuse, and I remind them that hypnosis works best, when they actually follow the advice of the hypnotist.

Experience has shown me that if a client puts in the effort to listen to the recording, he will actually feel better about reaching his goal. If he refuses to listen to it, he's probably rejecting all your other suggestions, and he shouldn't be surprised if he fails.

A smart hypnotist, would record her own Sleep Hypnosis recordings, that cover all of the most common client needs: Weight loss, stop smoking, confidence, overcoming grief, fears, reducing stress, etc. She would give these recordings away for free, on her website. She can offer anyone who downloads a free recording, a discount rate for online hypnosis. Great business marketing.

Using Hypnosis To Break Bad Habits

People are creatures of habit. All behavior is habitual, repeated over and over, almost automatically, whenever the need arises.

We call the area where all these habits are stored, like strings of code in a computer, the subconscious mind.

The subconscious mind instinctively accepts the status quo, and fears the unknown. Your basic instinct is to be "conservative", trusting things and people you already know, and fearing strangers and strange ideas.
Habits serve us well, because they are familiar ways of behaving, and give us expected results, with minimum mental effort.

The habit of driving a car is so automatic for us, that we don't actually remember every step in the process, we just kind of "oversee" the driving, while our subconscious mind completes a million different tasks, checking the mirrors, watching nearby cars, spotting a stop sign, and avoiding deer and pedestrians. Meanwhile, our conscious mind may be enjoying a song on the radio, chatting on the phone, or even texting!

Bad habits develop because we receive some benefit from the habit, at least initially. Usually, the habit serves a useful purpose, or it satisfies a need.

When we start smoking cigarettes, we are usually young. The cigarette makes us feel "relaxed", mature, and socially cool. And because we are young, the health consequences simply don't matter. For most of us, as teenagers, we simply don't understand what an addiction is, until we are caught in its web.

When the side effects of a habit are greater than any percieved benefit, we call this a BAD habit, because we don't want it anymore.

Bad Habits satisfy a need.

Usually, the habit develops as a way to manage stress, reduce anxiety, or to feel relaxed. People who smoke, drink, overeat, or abuse drugs are all "self-medicating" in order to feel better.

People who bite their nails, pick obsessively at their skin, pull their own hair out, crack their knuckles constantly, these cases probably developed in childhood, as a way to feel in control, or it could also be "attention-seeking behavior".

Very often, bad habits are caused, as a form of self-punishment. Self destructive habits, and self sabotage, are the result of unresolved feelings of guilt, shame, regret, or worthlessness.

Other bad habits are not physical in nature. Procrastination, depression, negative self-talk, obsessive-compulsive behavior, these bad habits can do enormous emotional damage, robbing a person of self-esteem and confidence, while pretending to protect a person from fears, failures, and disappointments.

Anatomy of a Bad Habit

Bad habits often develop in childhood. The child learns to copy the negative coping behavior of adults and other children. Children are sponges, absorbing information from those around them. It is impossible for a child to avoid the influence of the people nearest to him.

If a child sees his mom smoking cigarettes, and sees his dad drink till he's drunk and stupid, and sees his teenage brother taking prescription drugs to get high, there is a high likelihood the child will copy this behavior.

Usually, a bad habit starts out as an adequate way of dealing with stress and other negative emotions. When a teen starts smoking, there are almost no health risks (that comes much later in life). So, from the teenagers view, smoking is a good way to reduce stress. If you ask a teen about lung cancer, he will usually explain that he can quit anytime he wants, and he will definitely quit before his lungs and heart quit on him.

Most bad habits develop as a coping tool, for stress, fears, boredom, loneliness, or emotional pain.

Other bad habits simply make us feel good. People who love to get high fall into this group. Thrill seekers are people who get a "rush" from exciting and even dangerous behavior, like taboo sexual encounters, robbing a bank, and similar risky yet thrilling acts.

The negative effects of bad habits are many:

1. Low Self Esteem
2. Physical Health Problems (Smoking, Obesity)
3. Anxiety
4. Loneliness
5. Depression
6. Sexual Problems
7. Family Problems
8. Financial problems

How To Break a Bad Habit

The subconscious mind fears the unknown. For this reason, it clings to a bad habit, as something "familiar". It doesn't matter if the habit is dangerous, like smoking or overeating.

We need to find out what triggers the bad habit, and what needs are being satisfied with it.

Next, we need to find a replacement behavior, that satisfies the same need, but without any negative side effects.

Gum can replace cigarettes. Fresh fruit can replace sugary snacks.

Look for positive replacements that are connected to increased self-esteem, confidence, stress reduction, and improved health.

To break a bad habit, the client must really want to make the behavior change. He must believe that personal change is possible, and he must be willing to take the actionable steps his hypnotist recommends.

Hypnosis and Depression

I like to divide depression into 3 subsections:

    □□ *Broken Heart*-- A lover who feels she can't live without her "twin flame", her "soulmate."
    □□ *PTSD*-- The client may have been the victim of childhood abuse, sexual abuse, combat trauma, and battered wife.

☐☐ *Death of a Loved One*-- The clients' mother, child, or partner dies, and the grief is crushing her.

For clients with a broken heart, I begin with some chair therapy, in hypnosis of course. The client will be seated in front of the former lover, and start expressing her pain, by saying, "You hurt me so bad! You hurt me when...."

I encourage the client to "spill her guts", and unload on the former lover. Only when she is nakedly honest about the pain she feels, are we ready to proceed.

Next, I ask her to imagine that her former lover has sat there and heard everything she said to him. What might he say in response?

Usually, the former lover (speaking through the client), will say, "I never meant to hurt you. I'm sorry."

Now I ask the client if she is willing to forgive her former lover. I explain that forgiveness doesn't mean she approves of his behavior. It just means she is ready to let go of the pain attached to this event.

When she declares that she has forgiven her former lover, I clap my hands, literally, to make her feel good about this breakthrough.

I explain that she has begun the healing process, and the next step is to stop revisiting the old memories, the painful words, the hurt and the lies. Whenever her mind returns to those painful memories, she should remind herself that she forgave him. Her painful past is like a scab on her arm, in order for it to heal correctly, she needs to stop picking at it, and just leave it alone.

The easiest way to forget about a former lover, is to find a new lover.

I always push online dating, when a client has a broken heart.

Too often, a client feels like no one else would find her attractive or loveable. This is simply not true, and anyone who is not too selfish or picky can find love on a dating site.

I met my wife on a dating site, and I am as happy as I have ever been.

There are few alternatives to dating online. Going to a bar or nightclub is a bad move. Hitting on coworkers or people at church or the grocery store seems way more desperate and ineffective than online dating.

If your client doesn't find a new love interest soon, she will feel lonely, empty, and isolated. Then, when her former lover texts her for a booty call, she will accept, reasoning that no one else is interested in her.

For PTSD clients, the method is similar.

Instead of the former lover going in the chair, I ask the client to put "Whoever hurt you most in life."

The client accuses the person in the chair (the Accused) of hurting her, and we encourage high emotions, crying and shouting if appropriate.

I ask the client to imagine what reply the Accused would give, and it's usually that they were drunk, or too young, or too selfish to make better choices.

After forgiveness, I may ask the client to sit in the Chair herself, and ask if she needs to forgive herself for anything.

Like the Broken Heart script, I ask the client to "let go" of all this pain. Forgiveness means to let it all go, and to stop returning to those painful memories, so they can heal properly.

And finally we have the Death of a Loved One.

In this session, I have the "Loved One" sit in the chair. The client may wish to start by saying how the Loved One hurt them, if I have any reason to believe there was any abuse or neglect in their past.

I normally pretend that the client has one last chance, to say whatever is important to say, to this special person they love.

The client will cry, and as a hypnotist you should encourage tears, as a way to wash away the pain, and let these emotional wounds heal.

After the client has said everything she needs to say, I ask her to forgive the Loved One, then forgive herself.

Finally, I ask the client to dedicate their life, to the memory of the Loved One. If the Loved One is the client's mother, for example, I want the client to live in a way that will make the memory of their mother proud. This is important.

In all cases of depression, I ask the client to see themselves as a survivor, not as a victim. The client needs to be tough, because only the strong survive.

I also remind the client that even though she feels hurt, the universe is not picking on her. She is NOT being punished for anything. The world is a cruel, painful, dangerous place, and her pain and grief is something that everyone feels at some point in life. Everyone feels horrible the first time they get dumped by a boyfriend, or when a friend dies suddenly, or when an uncle gets creepy with them. It is easy to feel isolated and alone, but these tragedies happen to all of us, in different ways.

Sometimes, if the client feels too much pain, I might recommend a support group. These groups can help the client feel like she is not alone in her pain. Be careful though; some of these groups can be very negative, and might make your client feel worse.

Depression is never a 1 session fix. The client has to return for multiple sessions, to benefit from real healing.

I want to offer the client who suffers from grief a reality check. Everybody, from the beginning of time, has either lost someone they truly loved, or they died loveless and alone. Either way is horrible but everyone has to deal with loss. Everyone.

Sometimes a client may feel like their grief is exceptionally cruel or extraordinary difficult to deal with. As if their pain was somehow worse than someone else's and justifies all the extra crying and misery. That is not true.

I love my mother more than anyone ever loved anyone, and I am sure you feel the same way about your family. When we lose someone special, it hurts. But in order for us to survive as individuals and as a species, we have to set a time for grief and then a time for moving on.

One thing I like to do for the grief client, is give them direct suggestions, so that whenever they think of their Loved One, they choose to think of positive aspects only. Never anything negative or depressing. If there is not enough material in their memories for positive replacement of unhappy memories, I suggest that they create new memories, and imagine future interactions in Heaven or in some ideal Paradise where they will be with their loved one again, sharing and caring and loving.
In their mind, the fantasy of being reunited in a paradise situation with their loved one feels very pleasant and satisfying.

What if the client is experiencing chronic depression? If that's the situation, I prescribe a heaping dose of positivity. Depression is an extremely negative emotion. To counterbalance this destructive emotion, I recommend kindness, charity, volunteering, activism, and social love.

Maybe your depression client could make people smile by painting kindness rocks and leaving them in public areas for people to find. Maybe your client can volunteer at the animal shelter to help dogs and cats who have no one to love them.

Usually, I try to make the pain that the client feels a motivation to help other people who feel the same way. So, if a woman is sad because her child died from leukemia, I ask her to volunteer to help other mothers deal with the grief of losing a child. If a woman is raped, and that caused the depression, she can volunteer with support groups that will help other women cope with being victims of rape.

The most effective way of dealing with depression, in my opinion, is to get someone to do positive, generous, selfless actions that help others. A suicidal person is a very negative person. They feel that the world is unbearably cruel, and that their quest for happiness is an impossibility. I ask these clients to step out of their selfish bubble, and help people just like themselves, victims of cruelty, and somehow, magically, their own pain gets smaller, the more they help others.

I call this active love, because so many times we say we love animals or we say we love children, but we don't take any actions to help those who are suffering.

I feel that the best way to improve a depressed person's life, is to help them practice active love. They can take care of a dog, care for a cat, volunteer and help foster children, read stories to children in the Cancer Ward of the hospital, help a recovering addict get back on their feet, help a recently crippled boy learn to live with crutches and a wheelchair.

The tremendously positive and satisfying feeling these clients receive from stepping out of their selfishness and actively helping in a way that really makes a difference is the antidote for chronic depression and grief.

What about the client who is suffering from a broken heart? The client who got dumped on, or cheated on, or the client who is recently divorced?
The solution is simple and obvious. The client with the broken heart needs to begin dating again.

The rejected lover often feels they are unlovable, ugly, and unattractive. In a very real sense, they have hypnotized themselves into believing that they are unlovable. It is my job as hypnotist to make them feel comfortable about dating. I usually ask them to go on Plentyoffish.com because it has a large number of people therefore a greater likelihood of making a meaningful connection.

For the heartbroken client, I suggest they start with a headline on their dating profile that says "Friends First." This will filter out all the horny guys and players.

The great thing about online dating is, everyone has to be polite or they will be banned from the site. So if a jerk says something mean to a lady, she simply reports him and he is banished from the site. So the woman has the advantage on these sites. In fact, if 1000 men see a woman's profile, and 999 think she is ugly, but just one guy thinks she is attractive and worth getting to know, the woman doesn't see or notice the rejections because they are invisible. She will get one message from the guy who thinks she is attractive, and he will say something polite yet flirty, and that simple compliment will do more for her self-esteem than 100 hypnosis sessions.

Self Sabotage

The biggest reason people fail to reach their goals is self sabotage. They ruin their chance for success by failing to take actions they know are necessary for success. And if they do take action, it is half hearted or inconsistent.

Self sabotage is any behavior that impedes your success:

- *Limiting Beliefs*
- *Negative Self Talk*
- *Excuses*
- *Procrastination*
- *Fears*

It doesn't matter how much natural talent you have. You may be super creative, a true visionary. But the sad truth is, if you cannot overcome the destructive behaviors listed above, you will never reach your full potential.

I am just like you. For so many years, I sabotaged my own chances for success. That's why I'm a hypnotist today. I want to help others break this harmful habit of being your own worst enemy.

How do we stop self sabotage?

By increasing our self love.

I have to love myself enough, to push those limiting beliefs aside, and replace them with a belief in my own intelligence and ability to set a goal and reach it. By increasing my self love, I am slowly changing my narrative voice in my own head. The narrative voice that used to say, "You'll never make it, you aren't strong or smart enough" has to be replaced with, "I believe in myself, and I love myself."

If you don't love yourself fully, I want you to contact me, let's do a forgiveness session online, and find out why you don't love yourself. Once we heal all the pain, guilt, shame and regrets from your past, your self love will shine through, and make it easy to stop self sabotage.

You don't "Break" a bad habit, you "Replace" it

You need to have a plan, ahead of time, for how you are going to respond to stress without feeding your bad habit. For smokers, they can replace a cigarette with gum, hard candy, or breath mints. For dieters, they can replace sugary snacks with fresh fruit.

You should avoid as many triggers as possible. If you smoke when you drink, then don't drink. These 2 habits should be addressed together, as alcohol can impair your good judgement, so that it's hard to quit smoking when you are drunk.

You should join a "Quit Group", of people who have recently quit the same thing. Do you know why we like to quit "in private?"

It's because we don't want people to see us fail. By that logic, you should join a quit group, on Facebook, or Reddit, so you feel the motivation of the group, and you don't feel all alone. When someone else expects you to succeed, this has a powerful impact on your efforts.

You need to stay away from negative people. Anyone who is addicted to drugs, or is depressing, abusive or just plain difficult to like, should be avoided. You don't have to stop loving family members that are grumpy. But you do have to stay away from them, while you break your bad habit.

The reason for this is simple. When you argue or fight, or feel any negative emotions, your stress levels increase. When you feel high stress, you are likely to seek relief, by returning to the bad habit for comfort.

Additionally, you should be hanging around people you admire. People who have the qualities and values you want in your life. If you are quitting smoking, you should be associating with people you like, who do not smoke.

In hypnosis, I will ask the smoker to visualize himself, saying "NO" to someone who offers her a cigarette. She is going to imagine herself 5 years into the future, clean and healthy, smoke free and happy. These images help her to see herself as a nonsmoker, an essential step to quitting successfully.

When we break a bad habit, we might feel like we need to become an entirely new person.

Sometimes, we really do need to change big parts of our personality and behavior. I am thinking of drug abuse, sex addictions, and abusive relationships.

But other times, all we need to change, is the way we view the bad habit. You weren't born with this bad habit. You don't need to quit smoking, you just need to return to your previous nonsmoking life.

It is very important, that you overcome your negative self talk. To do this, use the word "but." For example, a smoker's negative self talk would go like this: "I'm going to die if I don't have a cigarette soon, **but** no one has ever died from not having a cigarette, so I know I'll be fine."

Let me tell you a secret: That negative self talk likes to pretend he's your friend, but if you actually recorded the advice, you would soon realize he's not your friend. He represents your fears, overblown, magnified, and he is sabotaging your success.

You need to make a plan for failure. Now I'm sure some hypnotists will say that creates an expectation of failure. But those same hypnotists do not like to talk about what percent of their clients actually stop smoking or lose weight.

It is unrealistic to assume that because I hypnotized you, and you went deep in trance, and I declared that you would never smoke again, that we are finished here.

I believe the most powerful hypnotist in your life, is that voice in your head, the narrative voice, the one you have silent conversations with, all the time, everyday.

Most of us have trouble even separating ourselves from that narrative voice in our heads. It has been there since we were children, and has never stopped worrying, fretting, accusing.

Most of hypnosis is designed to stop and redirect this inner narrative, to something positive, that can help break the bad habit.

So what if you screw up, and smoke a cigarette?

First, you should have a plan for this. Without a step by step plan, you will simply get discouraged and give up.

Here is your plan, if you screw up.

☐☐ **Promise Yourself You Will Not Give Up.** You are breaking a habit that you had for years. Don't be shocked if you screw up and sneak a smoke. As long as you don't give up on your goal, you will become a permanent nonsmoker.

☐☐ **Identify the Feeling that Made You Screw Up.** Did you feel stressed out? Bored? Angry? Sad?

☐☐ **How Will You Deal with This Feeling the Next Time?** If you feel stress, you can listen to some relaxing music...take a walk on a nature trail...go to the gym...MEDITATE....YOGA....

☐☐ **"I Will Reach My Goal."** Renew your motivation and commitment to succeed. Nothing has changed except your Quit Date. All your reasons for quitting still exist, right? Poor health, low self esteem, you need to realize that the only time you fail, is when you give up.

☐☐ **Ask for Help.** Set an appointment for hypnosis, to reinforce your motives for quitting. Join an online forum, on Facebook or Reddit, and talk to other people, who are going through the same thing. You are not alone in this.

Junkie Thinking

If I were to call a client a junkie, I would hurt them unnecessarily. Even if they are actually addicted to heroin, calling them a junkie would not help at all.

But when the junkie-type thoughts come up in a session, I am quick to label them junkie thinking.

No one likes to think of themselves as a junkie. The word brings images of someone stealing from their family, to pay for drugs...sunken veins and hypodermic syringes...jail, homelessness, and tragedy await the junkie.

I summon these images, that we all naturally detest, without labelling the client as a junkie.

For an overweight client, who claims she can't drive home from work without stopping for a snack, I would say "That's junkie thinking." She will recoil a bit at that statement. That is good. Push that snack out of your mind, because your heroin is in the shape of a candy bar or bag of Doritos.

For a smoker, the seeds of a relapse can start days before the actual relapse happens. The client might see a stranger on a park bench, "relaxing" with a cigarette. Her mind might say, "He gets to smoke, but I can't because I quit. AARRGH!"

These feelings of deprivation are what I call junkie thinking. This is why people screw up and relapse. Junkie thinking is a pestering, nagging thought that will grow over time, until you feel like you are making this huge and unreasonable sacrifice, by not smoking. Soon the person starts feeling sorry for herself, and starts obsessing about cigarettes.

Stop this self sabotage, this junkie thinking, by repeating to yourself that smoking has no value. Smoking is not going to make you happy. In fact, the longer you don't smoke, the happier and healthier you will feel.

"Romancing the cigarette" is dangerous. After you quit for a few days, it's easy to forget why you wanted to quit in the first place.

That's why I strongly recommend 4 sessions. Even if you successfully quit after the first session, we need to reinforce this success, and strengthen your motivation and commitment.

The additional sessions will focus on removing the junkie thinking:

- "I quit for 3 days, and it wasn't that difficult...I bet I could smoke for a few more days, and then quit again. No big deal."
- "I have an important meeting today, and I can't be distracted. I should smoke a cigarette, then quit after this meeting."
- "My boyfriend is being a jerk, why does he have to be so difficult when I'm trying to quit? It's his fault if I go back to smoking."

Like a woman in an abusive relationship, it's easy to remember all the good times you had with cigarettes, and ignore the bad times. We can remember how nice it was to relax after a big dinner, and smoke. We find it easy to forget all the shame that cigarettes have brought us. Have you ever asked a complete stranger if they have "an extra" cigarette? Did you ever run out of cigarettes, and start smoking "snipes", the last inch of an old discarded cigarette? Did you ever have to stand in the rain and snow, to smoke outside? Did your doctor ever make you feel stupid, for damaging your lungs and heart?

Why do we forget all the bad times with smoking, and only remember the good?

Junkie thinking.

In 72 hours, the nicotine will leave your body, but the habit of smoking still lingers. The mind is VERY creative, and if junkie thinking creeps in, your mind may sabotage your efforts to quit, nagging you, appealing to you, to smoke "just one cigarette."

These are all lies.

Junkies always lie, especially to themselves. There is never "just one cigarette." No such thing, ever.

Focus your attention on the Narrative Voice inside you. It's that voice that you constantly hear in your head, advising you, warning you, criticizing you, and criticizing others. Some counselors think this narrative voice is the voice of your primary parent, and you learned to listen to this voice as a small child.

Every time thoughts of smoking enters your mind, correct them. Never allow them to grow into an urge you can't control. Protect your Quit! Tackle and deflect thoughts of smoking, before they get a chance to grow.

If you screw up and smoke a cigarette, you gave in to junkie thinking. Don't let this happen. Don't ruin your quit.

But if you do screw up, here is what you do:

- *Stop smoking immediately. The worst possible thing to do is give up. Your deviously creative mind will probably try to trick you into postponing your quit for a few days. Don't listen to that junkie thinking! Stop smoking right away and get your mind focused on your ultimate goal—becoming a nonsmoker.*
- *Write out a list of reasons for quitting. This is important. This simple step brings the reality of quitting back into focus. If you have screwed up before, get out your list, read it over and over, and add something to it. This list represents your TRUE priorities, and it's super important to read them, out loud, often, to bring these priorities back into focus. Carry the list with you, and memorize it, burning the words into your memory, into your heart.*
- *Get Educated. Read lots of books about smoking, its damage to the body, and related topics. Now you can face these dangers armed with real knowledge. This will strengthen your commitment to quit.*
- *Get Support. Find people online and in person, that have a*

> *similar goal as you. Stop Smoking support groups are everywhere now, including on Facebook and Reddit. And Weight Loss groups are even easier to find than stop smoking groups.*

- ***One Day At A Time.*** *Just think about today. You can stay smoke-free just for today, right? That's all you need to do! Don't think about the past or the future, just focus on not smoking for today. Your power is right here, right now. You can't change what happened yesterday, and the best way to create a bright future, is by not smoking today. Keep is simple, and keep it in the present tense.*

- ***Accept Yourself.*** *We are all human. We all make mistakes. If you screwed up and smoked, it doesn't mean you are a failure. As long as you don't give up, you can't fail. Learn from what went wrong the previous times, and make corrections, so you avoid those same mistakes in the future.*

- ***Love Yourself.*** *Be kind to yourself. Be patient. Forgive yourself for past failures. Hypnosis can help with forgiveness. Learn to relax. Meditate. Practice Yoga. Do good for the people you love, and the social causes that are important to you. Be sure to pamper yourself with a reward, for every day you don't smoke. You deserve it!*

Don't "Fight" Junkie Thinking, Ignore It

In hypnosis, I often ask a client to imagine his arm is an iron bar that cannot bend. Then when I try to push his arm down, he pushes back with equal force.

This is exactly what happens when you push up against an intrusive thought, like the unwanted thought of smoking.

The thought carries its own resistance because of the emotional energy you grant it. The secret to breaking any bad habit is to have no emotional connection to the triggering thoughts at all.

We do this by desensitizing the client through repeated age regression or visualization so that the client completely neutralizes any emotional impact from the offending thoughts.

The emotion behind a smoker's urges is fear.

There is a fear of quitting. So when the urge, which is a thought, pokes its head up, it is attached and connected to a fear emotion. We can use exposure therapy to visualize clients rejecting the thought of smoking correctly.

You are the commander of your own mind. Thoughts serve you, not vice versa. When an unwanted thought, like the urge to smoke, enters your mind, observe it, without accepting it.

Imagine you are laying on your back, in a beautiful summer meadow. Staring up at the sky, you watch the white puffy clouds, as they move slowly across the sky. Now, imagine those clouds are your thoughts. They float into your mind, and you observe them, but you don't accept them, you don't feed them with your mental attention. You just watch them drift out the other side of your mind, while you smile and laugh, and wonder how it became so easy to disengage your awareness from your thoughts!

Fear is never rewarded. Courage is.

Hypnosis and Beliefs

Hypnosis is all about belief systems and changing erroneous beliefs, and suggesting better things to believe, healthier things. I can honestly say that I've been fascinated by the things that people believed in from ancient times and modern times. Cults have always fascinated me and so have the major religions.

All my life I always felt like I was waiting to find that one religion that made sense to me, that spoke to me in a personal way, one that sparked a light in my soul, and said, "You belong here Alex."

I think the one big problem I had with religions was that we were always expected to accept whatever fate threw at us, when it came to our path in life and our circumstances.

This depressed me because I saw Catholics and Methodists, both praying for solutions to deeply painful problems in their lives, and when the solution never came, they frequently lost hope.

This is why I see hypnosis as the belief system of the future. In hypnosis my beliefs serve me. But in religion, I serve my beliefs. And so when I see a man who is afraid to leave his house, if I am a religionist I tell him, "Brother I will pray for you." But I am a hypnotist, so I say, "Brother I will hypnotize you, and you will get up and walk out of your house today."

Hypnosis is part Magic and part Hope...there is a Magic inside you, the source of all miracles, and I'm going to guide you to it.

When someone calls me and they have been smoking for 40 years, they feel like they are in a prison of hopelessness. And when they successfully quit smoking through hypnosis it is the most miraculous event to behold.

When we think of modern religions, we do not think of a place where Miracles routinely occur. Miracles are like lottery tickets in that they are exceedingly rare. But with hypnosis we can stack the deck in our favor, and increase the odds of us finding that miraculous ability, to change our behavior and our beliefs, and enhance the quality of our lives.

I believe that religions today are 99% Dogma and 1% miracles. And hypnosis is the exact opposite. Hypnosis is 99% miracles and 1% Dogma.

I believe that in the future, people will be able to exchange their old and outdated beliefs for more powerful and healthy beliefs, as easily as we exchange a pair of shoes. I believe that in the future, hypnosis will be used to heal every sort of emotional and mental pain, break every type of bad habit, and install powerful beliefs of self confidence and fantastic personal capabilities.

The belief system of the future is here today and it is called hypnosis.

I want you to email me for a free hypnosis session. We will talk about your goals and how hypnosis can help you. Video hypnosis is easy now with Skype and Facebook Messenger. I can hypnotize you in the privacy of your own home at a day and time that is perfect for you. I could charge you, but I want to make it easy for you to take the next step and improve your life dramatically. If you want to donate something to me after you reach your goal, that's great.

I am the only hypnotist that guarantees you will reach your goal after four sessions with me or your money back. Amazingly, no one has ever asked for a refund!

Let this be the day you take action towards improving your life in a big way. Email me, Alex the Hypnotist, FunWithHypnosis@gmail.com

3 Handshake Induction

- Hold her hand...point at your right eye with your left index, and ask her to focus on the spot just under your right eye.

- *"The first time I shake your hand, your eyes will start to feel tired."* (slightly shake their hand)

- *"The second time I shake your hand, you will want to close your eyes, but just keep your eyes focused on that spot under my right eye."*
- *"The third time I shake your hand, your eyes will close, and you will go into hypnosis."*
- 1 shake (*"your eyes are getting tired"*) 2 shake (*"keep your eyes on that spot"*) 3 shake (*"close your eyes and sleep"*)
- Immediately begin saying the relaxing patter phrases in the next chapter, to keep the client in trance.

Patter

All you need to help someone quit smoking or lose weight, is the scripts in the back of this book, and this section of "patter." Patter is a collection of a hypnotists favorite phrases, metaphors, and suggestions, that are memorized by constant practice, so they flow so naturally, the client accepts the words easily. Most patter is designed to increase relaxation, but others will help you control the pace of the session, and guide the client correctly.

Study the patter, then read the 2 scripts in the back of the book, and you will be ready to hypnotize a volunteer, to quit smoking or lose weight.

I want you to succeed! If you have any questions, email me, FunWithHypnosis@gmail.com

- Don't get stuck in the Narrative Thought Stream
- Every single outside sound will take you deeper
- The more your eyelids flitter, the deeper you will go
- All your inhibitions disappear, and you feel confident
- You need to tame your mind, and tame your passions, with yoga and meditation
- Can you put your feet flat on the floor for me? Can you put your hands on your lap for me?
- Take off your mask, and let your barriers down, so we can see the real you, the deeper you
- That's right, they are already moving closer. In a moment when your fingers touch, you can allow your eyes to close.
- I want a short description of the history of the problem.
- Most of your problems are emotional problems.
- If I knew then, what I know now
- What gives meaning to your life? What is important to you?
- The Inner Child loves to laugh and play
- Focus like a laser beam
- Smoking is now part of your ancient history

PLR (Past Life Regression) Patter

- Tell me more
- Look around you, what do you see?
- See yourself walking towards that waterfall, what do you notice?
- Hmm Hmmm
- Yes
- Tell me more about that. What's unusual about it?
- Can you elaborate on that?

- Mmm Hmmm
- How do you feel?
- OK
- What impressions are you getting?
- Keep exploring, and tell me what you find
- Now breathe out, letting the air and all your worries evacuate
- When reality matches our expectations, we feel happy
- Exhale, and feel how relaxed you already have become
- Let your consciousness fall away
- Frown lines in your face have disappeared, and your whole back has become looser and more comfortable
- Your breathing is deeper, and much more relaxed
- Inhale, and feel the peacefulness all around you
- Exhale, and find peace at the end of each breath, when your lungs and body are still
- Now I want you to Shout these statements, powerfully but silently, in your mind, so every corner of your mind accepts the statement
- How can we remedy this?
- Meditate on the pain itself. Notice every detail about it. When does it come, how long does it stay? Throbbing, or piercing? On a level of 1 to 10, how strong? Imagine yourself, stepping backwards, away from the pain, and seeing from far away. So far, you can barely see it.
- That little girl is still alive. In fact I'm looking at her right now.
- Breathe In Deeply. Exhale Fully.
- You feel wonderfully relaxed. So deeply relaxed.
- You feel a wonderful sense of deep relaxation.
- There is NOTHING between the numbers 5 and 7, if you try to find anything between 5 and 7 you will find that your mouth will totally lock down and shut, there is NOTHING between the numbers 5 and 7.

(Eye Lock Convincer)

> "Take your right index finger,
> and place it at the center top of your head,
> now close your eyes,
> I want you to imagine that your head is invisible, and
> you can see your finger from inside your head,
> you are looking through the top of your head,
> and you can see your finger...
> Can you see it?
> Good,
> As you look up at your own finger,
> you will be unable to open your eyes...
> Go ahead and try to open them,
> they will not open...
> Good, you can stop trying,
> and keep your eyes closed."

- You feel Groggy, Drowsy, Sleepy. You will go into a beautiful deep state of natural sleep.
- You can hear me but you won't wake up.
- The more intense emotions you feel, the more suggestible you are.
- Everyday is better than the day before.
- A person's greatest fear is not being loved by others.
- I want you to think of the deepest level of sleep you have ever felt, and then automatically let yourself feel the same way now.
- Now let's see if you will allow yourself to go even deeper.
- The more you try to open your eyes, the tighter they become, locking down even tighter.

- You can hear me but you won't wake up.
- You will be able to talk to me, and tell me things that you never could say when you were awake.
- When I snap my fingers you will be 10 years old.
- Listen carefully. Every time I touch my nose, you will

fall into a deep sleep. You will not remember this con-
versation. When I count to 3 you will open your eyes.
1,2,3 (then touch your nose, and if he doesn't go to sleep,
you must re-induct him)

- Let yourself fall into a deep, sound, sleep, just like when
  you sleep at night, only deeper.
- Let my suggestions in your mind without being ana-
  lyzed.
- Comfortably, calmly, quietly, and quickly
- Don't help me lift your hand up, let it remain loose, limp,
  and relaxed.
- Simply follow my basic instructions instantly.
- If you have average intelligence, and you can follow
  basic instructions, you can be hypnotized.
- Think about relaxing, and doing everything I ask you to
  do, it's easy.

- Let's make an agreement, I am here to help you. In order
  to help you, you have to do everything I ask instantly.
  We are going to focus your concentration, and we are
  going to turn that concentration into a deep, pleasant
  relaxation.
- When I touch your shoulder, your head will drop down,
  but you will remain supported in your chair.
- When I lift up your hand don't help me just let it relax.
- "Let a smile grow on your face right now, as you think
  of reaching your goals, this smile represents your true
  trust and belief in yourself, you can't hold this smile
  back, even if you wanted to."

- Close your eyes, and focus on your breathing. When you
  take a big breath, just nod your head for me.
- I want you to take your conscious mind, and put it in the
  corner.
- I want you to lift your right hand, this hand represents
  your confidence, let it go higher and higher, your confi-

dence is going higher and higher.
- Relax that jaw, let your mouth drop open, give yourself permission to relax that jaw, let your mouth drop open.
- Feeling safe, calm, secure, peaceful.
- Don't analyze, do everything I ask immediately, without thinking...
- Give yourself permission to relax even further.
- I want you to do everything I ask you to do quickly and without thinking.
- Just do everything that I ask instantly.
- You're doing perfect.
- Lighter and higher, lighter and higher, your hand and arm are floating, rising, lifting, faster now.
- When I emerge you from hypnosis, you will have a wonderful smile on your face that you cannot control, the more you notice your big smile the better it will feel, it will spread and spread until you are laughing, and feeling so happy. 1,2,3,4,5 Eyes open, wide awake.
- You are going to have a nice, restful sleep tonight. And sometime tonight, your subconscious mind is going to tell you what you need to do, in order to have a happy life.

- The sound of my voice, the touch of my hand, just helps you to relax even further.
- You are beginning to feel lighter, lighter and lighter. And your right hand, feels lightest of all.
- Take a nice deep breath, fill up your lungs, and SLEEP!
- In a moment I'm going to ask you to open your eyes. But instead of waking up, you will feel even more relaxed with your eyes open! When I touch your shoulder, just close your eyes, and let yourself drop even further into relaxation.
- You will go deeper into relaxation, not because I say so, but because it's natural for the human mind, to want to relax as fully as possible, because it's so enjoyable.

- There is no bottom to relaxation. You can always go deeper.

- Your world is going to be light, and bright.
- On the count of 3, let your eyes open and become fully alert. When they do, everything will seem a little bit better for you, and you will feel better than before.
- Notice a new energy in you, you feel like you are bathed in a cool mountain stream, you feel so fresh and exciting.
- Take a nice long deep breath, fill up your lungs and hold it. Now exhale and as you do, just let your eyes close naturally.
- When you KNOW you've relaxed your eyes so deeply that they will not work, TEST them, and try to open them, and you will see that they will not work.
- Time for you to truly relax, in your own special way.
- Go all the way down, to your own basement level, of your subconscious.
- Your hand is rising. Don't assist it, and don't resist it, just let it happen naturally. Enjoy that hand rising. More and more.
- The mind becomes flexible. You think of things, that you never thought of before.
- Think of Home. You are happy, at home...happy, at home...is home a happy place for you?

- I want you to hang onto every word I say, and accept my truth as reality.
- FEEL yourself relax deeper.
- I want you to realize that the number 2 has vanished from your memory banks.
- Nod your head if you understand.
- When I tap you on the forehead, you are going to be Joyce. OK, Joyce, you heard what he said, now respond to him.

- You have magnets on the center of your palms, you can feel it.
- Just relax, Go Inside, deeper, deeper, deeper.
- When I say 1,2, Wide Awake, your eyes will open, you'll be ready to respond to the suggestions I have given, and you will be ready to be hypnotized. Nod your head if you understand.
- Enjoy this experience, of drifting through your own powerful imagination.
- OK, now follow that feeling back to the first time you ever felt that way. 3,2,1 be there now. Is it daytime or nightime?

- I want you to go back as far as you need to go, to where your weight problem first began.
- Let that feeling of strength, of unstoppability, grow inside you.
- Today, this week, and for all the rest of your life.
- You made a POWERFUL decision today. A decision to take back control of a part of your life.

- In a moment, I'm going to touch your hand, and it will start to lift. It's going to get lighter and lighter, and float towards your face.
- It's starting to lift now, fingers are twitching, lighter and lighter, faster now, lifting up towards your face. You're doing brilliantly.
- You are safe and relaxed. Your legs will support you.
- Your head is feeling heavy. Your shoulders are relaxing.
- That's right, your eyes are flickering, going deeper.

- As I rock your shoulder you will continue to relax. As I rock your shoulder you can feel your head relaxing and your neck relaxing further.
- In a moment I'm going to touch the back of your hand, and it's going to start lifting up towards your face. Just

like it's being pulled up on an invisible wire.
- Now as I touch the back of your hand, it's going to feel lighter and lighter.
- When you sit down to have your meal, you will close your eyes, and say, "One Half". When you say the words "One Half," you will magically feel full after only eating half the food on your plate. You will not want to finish your food, because you will feel so wonderful and full, and if you were to continue eating, you would only feel stuffed and uncomfortable.

- You're going to find that the weight loss comes easily and effortlessly for you. The pounds will just drop off.

Jerry Kein Induction--

Take a nice long deep breath, and hold it.
Now exhale and close your eyes down.
Put your awareness on your eyelids, and relax them
completely, so they just won't work.
And when you done this go ahead and give them a little test.
Now take the same feeling that you have in your eyelids, and
bring it from the top of your head, to the tips of your toes.
Let your whole body relax.
Now let's deepen this relaxation.
In a moment I will ask you to open and close your eyes.
When you close your eyes, you will let your phys-
ical body become much more relaxed.
Open your eyes.
Close your eyes.

That's good, go all the way down...

In a moment I will ask you to open and close your eyes again.
This time, just double the feeling of relaxation.

Open your eyes. Close your eyes.

Now let's find out if we have all the relaxation we need. In a moment I'm going to raise your hand and drop it, and when it drops back into your lap, it'll just plop there, and when it plops down just let yourself relax much deeper. Don't help me lift, let me do all the lifting.

OK, we have the body relaxed, now let's relax the mind.
In a moment you will begin counting backward starting from 100.
After every number, you will say, "Deeper Sleep".
After a few numbers, it doesn't take long, your mind will relax so completely, the numbers will fall from your mind, they will drop from your mind, and when that happens, just stop counting and relax even further.
All you have to do is want that to happen and it'll be there for you.

Begin counting now.

Relax the numbers right out of your mind.

Let the numbers fade from your mind.

Good. The mind is relaxed, your body is relaxed.

Age Regression Patter--

- *I want you to know that you can relive any part of your life. Everything we've ever done is stored within our minds.*
- *You can relive any part of your life, that you want to live.*
- *You live a life of reflected action, and you can remember anything you want.*
- *I want to to think back, to when you were a little girl. Think of a time when you were having so much fun. It could have been a birthday party, or a Christmas morning, as long as it was a wonderful, wonderful time.*
- *I'm going to count back from 3 to 1, and you will go back to that special time, when you were having so much fun.*
- *3 .2 .1 .*

More Patter:

- I'm going to pick your hand up and drop it, and when I do, all your presents will be open, and you can tell me which present you like the best.
- Let that scene fade, and that happy memory will stay with you forever.
- When I count from 1 to 3, you will drift back even further in time and space, further back in your mind, when I drop your hand you will be there.

- By what name should I call you.
- I'm going to lift this hand and when I drop it you will feel wonderful.

- Leave that fear back in the past, where it belongs.
- You've punished yourself long enough.
- From this moment on, the more frightened and scared you feel, the more calm and relaxed you will become. What used to frighten you will now make you feel so calm. Doesn't that sound wonderful?

Street Hypnosis--

- "You look like you like to have fun, I'm Alex, I'm a hypnotist, would you like to play some mind games?"
- Can you stand over here? Can you hold your hands straight out? Can you interlock your fingers? Can you hold out your index fingers, about an inch apart? Good.
- Where your Attention goes, Energy flows.
- (C.I.Q....Compliment, Introduction, Question) "Hi, I like your smile, I'm Alex, I'm a hypnotist, have you ever been hypnotized?"

Standard Phrases for Induction--

- "The deeper you go the better you will feel, and the better you feel, the deeper you will go to sleep."
- "With every breath you take, every noise you hear, every word I say and every thought that you think, you'll go deeper and deeper to sleep."
- "Every muscle in your body from the tips of your toes to the tips of your fingers, now becoming so limp, so loose and so relaxed."
- "Each and every muscle in your body, now becoming so heavy and so tired."
- "Your eyelids are feeling so heavy and so tired, in fact, the harder you try to keep them open, the more they want to close tightly, as you relax completely."
- "As you sit (or lie) there in the comfortable chair, it almost feels as though every movement would be a great effort, as though you are sinking down deeply into the chair and into calm, satisfying, relaxation."
- "This feeling of warmth and relaxation, is now travelling around your entire body and as you continue to breathe deeply and regularly, you are drifting deeper and deeper to sleep."
- "All the worries, stresses and tensions of days gone by, are leaving your mind and leaving your body now, allowing you to relax completely."
- "In a few moments, when I awake you, you'll have an overwhelming desire to do almost everything I say, you'll find that you'll enjoy living your part in tonight's show to the full, and will carry out all that I suggest, as an automatic reflex action."
- "Just as your subconscious makes you breathe at night, or circulates the blood around your body, in just the same way you can faithfully rely upon your subconscious mind to help you eliminate this problem from your every day life."
- "It becomes habit in your subconscious mind to smoke

(or whatever) and now your subconscious mind will make it habit not to smoke (or whatever)"

- "Something that you thought would be difficult to achieve, will turn out to be ridiculously easy to do."
- "Each morning when you awake, from this moment forward, you will awaken with an inner warm glow of confidence, a renewed optimism to life and a more positive attitude to get things done."
- "Every day, in every way, things will be getting better and so much easier to cope with."
- "You have made a promise to yourself to (whatever) and while it may be alright, on occasion, to break a promise to a friend, your subconscious mind will not allow you to break a promise to yourself and, as such, success is guaranteed."

- Hypnosis is far too important to take seriously.
- Sleep. Close your eyes. Deeper and Deeper. As I rock your shoulder, you can continue to relax. Every word I say, every breath you take, every outside sound will take you into a more relaxed state of mind, and everything I say will become your reality. In a moment I'm going to touch the back of your hand, and it's going to lift, it's going to float up in the air towards your face.
- Your Mind Is Your Friend
- This will be a blissful feeling, more profound than anything you've felt before.

- "Whenever I say SLEEP or SLEEP NOW, you will return to this deep state of relaxation.
- "Sounds in the distance are mattering less and less."
- "Let yourself go deeper into yourself. Double the relaxation as your eyes close. Going deeper into the wonderful world that is hypnosis."
- "To help your mind experience the wonderful benefits of hypnosis, I'm going to ask you to count backwards

from 100, like this: 100, Deeper Sleep, 99, Deeper Sleep, 98, Deeper Sleep....

- "Can you imagine making a fist so tight, that it will not open? Now tell me, can you imagine the opposite? Can you imagine a hand so relaxed, that it will not move at all, no matter what? Well, that's the level of relaxation I want you to experience in hypnosis."
- "Hold onto the relaxation and stay in control by keeping your eyes closed."
- "Sink way down, relaxed, way, way, down."
- "And that makes you feel?"
- "All feelings are short lived unless we resist feeling them."
- "And how does that make you feel? Do you want to hold onto the feeling or release it?"
- "I want you to repeat after me. I feel better. I am allowed to feel better. I deserve to live a life free of fear. I can be happy anywhere in the world."
- "I'm going to show you how you can relax your mind even more."
- "With every sound that you hear, you will drift down deeper and deeper into relaxation."
- "The more you relax, the better you feel, the better you feel, the deeper you go. Deeper, deeper, deeper"
- "In a moment your fingers will touch."
- "Good, that shows you can concentrate."
- "Have you ever been hypnotized? Just place your feet together for me. Are you happy to be hypnotized? Let me just show you how it works, I'm gonna give you some instructions, just hold your hands out together like this."
- "This is a test on how well you can follow my suggestions."
- "Sleep, sleep and stand, your legs will support you."
- "Pull your fingers an inch apart, and stare at the gap

between your fingers, because in a moment your fingers will touch."

- "Sleep and stand, your legs will support you."
- "Are you left handed or right handed? Can I borrow your arm?"

- "Close your eyes, Sleep, relax, deeper and deeper. Just sleep, all the way down, relaxing, just let my words become your reality."
- "Look at your hand, look at the lines on it, look at one spot."
- "As your hand begins to move toward your face, your eyes will change focus, and when you become aware of your eyes, close your eyes, and SLEEP."
- "In a moment, I'll say, "1,2, wide awake" and when I do your eyes will open, and you'll be wide awake and ready to be hypnotized."
- "When I count to 3, you will be wide awake, but you won't be able to remember your name. When I ask you what your name is, you won't remember, and you will think this is so funny, you will laugh out loud."
- "Hypnosis works best with people that are really creative, and have a high I.Q. These people are able to imagine my suggestions and allow them to become their reality"
- "Find your own balance as you go deeper into trance."
- "Bend your elbows like you're making a desperate prayer. Now spread your index fingers about an inch apart and stare at the gap between your fingers, because in a moment your fingers will touch. That's right, and when they touch, allow your eyes to close. SLEEP, that's right, deeper, deeper, deeper."
- "If at any point you feel that it's not working, just PRETEND that it's working. Just imagine that you are really hypnotized, and you are following all my suggestions perfectly."

- "Does everyone on stage WANT to be hypnotized? Good. Now here's what's going to happen. Hypnosis feels like you're half awake, half asleep. You'll hear my voice at all times. The fact is you may know what's going on all around you, you just don't care. Now the biggest secret about hypnosis is, never try to make it happen, just let it happen, it's like trying to fall asleep, the more you try, you just keep tossing and turning, but the moment you stop trying, you quickly fall asleep. Now hypnosis is very relaxing, let yourself just enjoy the ride."
- "You can and will follow my suggestions exactly, because you like to have fun."

- "That's fine, you're doing perfectly."
- "Just take a deep breath, and on the exhale, I want you to say out loud, "Relaxing Now""
- "Look at me, do not look away. Do exactly as I say, as I give you a suggestion. I'm going to take great care of you."
- "The more you try, you will realize there's nothing you can do, say or think to get your hands open, the more you try the harder they lock, tighter and tighter. Make the attempt, satisfy yourself, OK, stop trying."

- "Every breath you take. Every word I say. Every sound you hear, will take you deeper into trance."
- "This is the induction part, those in the audience can just sit back and relax, if you want to follow along that's great."
- "Please refrain from side conversations as we want everyone to be able to hear what's going on, but when it comes to laughter and applause go crazy, because that helps the people in trance feel comfortable."
- "Have you been hypnotized before? Great, all you have to do is just let yourself go, let me do all the work, just relax, do you like to relax? This is going to be so relaxing,

just let yourself go, free yourself to follow my suggestions."
- "What do you want to change today?"
- "Sleep. Relax. Let Go."
- "Locking down, squeezing tighter, you can't open them, squeeze them tight on the count of 3, so tight even I can't open them, you can't open them, tighter now, locking down, squeeze tighter, you can try to open them but you can't open them, try harder they won't open, 1, 2, when I count to 3 they will be tighter still, try really hard now, take a deep breath, and on 3 , 1,2,3 DEEP SLEEP, relaxing now loose, as I count down from 5 to 1, let every breath every thought relax you, let your mind and body relax, let yourself go deeper, 5, go 20 times deeper, limp and relaxed, as I touch your body, 4, mind and body melting now, you can follow ALL my suggestions now, 3, every breath, every beat of your heart takes you deeper, mind, body and soul relaxing deeper, free yourself to relax even deeper, let your arms hang limp, for the rest of the day, you have permission, to instantly fall into trance, you have the gift of entering trance easily, instantly."
- "Can you follow my suggestions for the next 3 minutes?"
- "When you are sure your eyes are locked down, shut as tight as they can, give them a little test, try to open them, you can't. Now lock them down even tighter, so tight even I can't open them. Try really hard to open them, you can't, they lock down even more."

- "Your hands are stuck together, try to open them, you can't."
- "If your hands are stuck together and you had some fun you can come up and join us onstage."
- "Yes?" "Does this work for you?" "Is everyone happy about this?"
- "1, 2, wide awake!"
- "Go into that place of hypnosis, into that place where

imagination expands."

- "Give me your hand. Take a deep breath for me, and SLEEP, now go deeper, and deeper, every nerve, every fiber, every muscle in your body is relaxing."
- "Deep asleep, deeper deeper, feeling fantastic, deep asleep."
- "In a moment I'm going to put my finger on your forehead, and when I put my finger on your head your eyes will close and you will go into a deep state of hypnosis."
- From this moment on everything I say will become your reality, because you have a super-powerful mind."
- "I'm going to count to 3, when I get to 3 you will awake, alert, feeling good, everything normal, 1,2,3 and WAKE."
- "Everyone give him a massive round of applause, he was brave for coming up here."
- "Are you left handed or right handed? Good, can I borrow your arm?"
- "No outside sound is important, just the sound of my voice."
- "Nod your head if you understand."
- "When I snap my fingers you will be back in the room wide awake."
- "Deeper, deeper, drifting down."
- "Everything back to normal."
- "In a moment, I'm going to borrow your arm, is that OK?" (point to it)
- "As you look at your hand, I want you to focus on just one spot."
- "As that hand starts to move toward face." (I'm moving it until it moves on its own)
- "As that hand starts to move toward face, your eyes WILL begin to change focus..." (statement of fact...pacing statement)
- "As you become aware of your eyes, CLOSE your eyes, and SLEEP, (snap fingers) and deeper, deeper drifting down, into a wonderful place of absolute bliss"

- "Everytime I click my fingers, it will get 10 times deeper."
- "When I count to 3, you will be eyes open, wide awake, 1,2,3"

- "Palms together, elbows bent like you're making a desperate prayer."
- "I want you to focus on the gap between your fingers, because in a moment they are going to come together and touch, just like two magnets getting closer and closer, they are already starting to go, you can feel them getting closer, almost there, the pull is getting stronger, you are doing brilliantly."
- "And when they touch, you can just allow yourself to close your eyes. When your fingers touch, your eyes will close."
- "Excellent, that shows you can concentrate, now I'm going to ask you to close your eyes concentrate in the same way, using your imagination."
- "Can you just sit back in your chair? Can you please put your feet on the floor?"

- Let those eyes open now, and notice how good you feel.
- All negative memories of your past are nothing but flickering images, they have no reality. They can no longer disturb you.
- Is there anything else that hasn't been done, that needs to be done, to eradicate this fear?
- I want you to TRY to find the fear in your mind. TRY hard to find the fear. The harder you try, the calmer and more relaxed you feel, because the fear is gone, you can't find it, because it's no longer there.

- "Imagine there is a string tied to your wrist, attached to 5 colorful helium balloons. Feel your hand starting to rise in the air, higher and higher, floating, rising, feeling

light as a feather."
- "These are happy balloons, so the higher they go, the better you feel."
- Your arm is rising high above your head, and now it is as stiff as a steel rod, you cannot bend it, the more you try to bend it the harder and stiffer it becomes, go ahead and try to bend it, you cannot."
- "When I count from 0 to 3, your arm will drop like a stone to your lap, and you will go twice as deep into relaxation. 0,1,2,3"

Magnetic Hands Induction--

- Hold your hands straight out. Hold them a foot apart.
- Stare at the gap between your hands, and begin to feel a magnetic pull, pulling your hands together.
- The more you stare at the space between your hands, the more the magnetic hands will pull your hands closer and closer together.
- That's the power of your subconscious mind, working to pull your hands together.
- Don't resist or comply, but the more you stare at the space between your hands, the more that magnetic pull will pull your hands together. Just let the subconscious mind do all the work for you.
- With every breath you take, your hands are being pulled closer and closer.
- Feel the magnetic pull getting stronger and stronger.
- As soon as your hands touch, just go ahead and close your eyes, and go into a deep sleep.
- Going down more, and more, more and more.
- Draw your attention to your breathing.

- The arm and hand is rising, faster and faster, light as a feather, towards your face.

- In a moment you will notice that your breathing is changing, becoming slow and regular, shake your head yes when you feel that.
- Your arm and your hand will have a tendency to feel lighter and lighter, shake your head yes when you feel that.
- Your arm and your hand is feeling lighter and lighter, lifting up, floating up, higher and higher, towards your face.

- The feeling is spreading, through your shoulders now, and your neck, and your solar plexus.
- I'm going to pick up the arm, and all the tension from the body is going to be collected in this arm. And when I drop the arm, all the tension is going to disappear.
- I'm going to count from 5 to 0, and when I count to 0, your arm will be as stiff as a bar of iron.
- Can you feel the bar now?
- You are changing your unconscious script. You are successful NOW, in this moment. Your success will grow, day after day. Your thoughts and ideas are moving towards your success, you are winning.
- A thought is going to start penetrating the mind.
- You have been fighting a frustration, for many years. That frustration is over. If your subconscious mind agrees, your index finger will rise.
- A smile grows on your face, a contagious smile that you can't control, it grows bigger and bigger, go ahead and try to stop it, you cannot.
- Open your eyes, and see your hand stuck to your face. It's funny, isn't it?
- <<<<<<<<<<<<<<<<

Stop Smoking Script

(You have just spent days reading my book about hypnosis. Now you can use this script to hypnotize someone who wants to quit smoking. Words in regular print are instructions, words in italics are spoken to the client. You should pepper your hypnosis session with LOTS of suggestions from my chapter in this book, "Patter". I want you to succeed, so if you have any questions at all, just email me and I will help you. FunWithHypnosis@gmail.com)

1. Ask Client to take a deep breathe, and close her eyes.

2. (Arm Heaviness Convincer) Ask her to raise her right arm straight up above her head, with her right fist closed tightly. *I want you to imagine you are holding a heavy bag, filled with sand. This bag is a brown canvas bag, and it's full of sand. This bag weighs over 10 pounds. Imagine what it feels like, to hold this heavy bag filled with sand high above your head. Can you see this bag in your mind's eye? Good. Imagine the weight of this bag of sand, pulling down on your arm as you strain to hold it. Can you feel the tension in the muscles of your shoulder, arm, and in the tiny muscles of your hand and fingers? Good, you are doing perfectly. When I count to 3 your arm will drop safely to your side, and you will enter a deep sleep. 1,2,3, your arm is now safely at your side, and you feel a deep relaxation.*

3. (Eye Lock Convincer) *I want you to focus your attention on the tiny muscles around your eyes. Focus all your attention on your eyelids, and give them permission to relax completely. It helps if you imagine that your eyelids are also heavy bags filled with sand. Allow your eyelids to relax so much, that they will not open. And when you are sure you've relaxed them so much, that they will not open, go ahead and give them a little test, and you will see that they will not open.* (Wait for 2

seconds) *Good, you can stop trying and keep your eyelids closed, and let yourself relax completely.*

4. *Let this relaxing feeling in your eyelids spread to the other muscles in your face, softening your expression, gently releasing any pockets of tension, in your neck and throat. Your shoulders are dropping now, slipping into a sleepy posture, and your arms are loose, limp, and relaxed, so comfortable and sleepy.*

5. *Your breathing is slow and regular, like the breathing of a sleeping person. Hypnosis is just like sleep, except you will always be able to hear my voice, and respond to my words. Your heart is beating softer, and a heavy sleepy feeling is spreading to every part of your body.*

6. (Fractionation) *In a moment I will ask you to open your eyes, and find a spot on the ceiling to stare at. You can choose any spot that suits you. Then I will ask you to close your eyes. Are you ready? OK, open your eyes and find a spot on the ceiling to stare at. Focus all your attention on that spot, ignoring any other distractions, blocking out all sensations. Now close your eyes, and feel yourself drifting deeper into sleepy relaxation.* (Do this 3 times)

7. (Look at your client. If she seems deeply relaxed, skip step 8)

8. (Losing the Numbers) *In a moment I'm going to ask you to count backward from 100. But you will count in a special way. You will count like this, "100, deeper sleep, 99, deeper sleep, 98, deeper sleep," and so on. But these numbers are special, because very soon they will drop out of your mind, fade away, and disappear. When that happens, just stop counting, and relax. Are you ready to begin? Good. Start counting backwards for me now.* (Every number she counts, you say things like, "Slower...Softer....Sleep is coming....The numbers are fading....The numbers are gone...." When she makes a long pause, or stops completely, say, "The numbers have dropped from your mind, you can stop counting and relax.")

9. (Arm Float Convincer) *I am speaking to your subconscious mind now, to your inner mind. As you think about your desire to stop smoking, your right arm is going to start to rise, float, levitate straight up towards the ceiling. The more intensely you desire*

freedom from cigarettes, the faster your right arm will rise, the higher it will rise. Don't assist it and don't resist it, just let it happen naturally, as you focus all your attention on breaking free from the poison of nicotine. Imagine all the wonderful things you can do, without health problems of any kind to slow you down. And as your right arm rises higher and higher, your inner mind is declaring the same desire, for an end to the shame of smoking, and its emotional pain. (Keep suggesting the phrases in this step, until the arm rises high. I like to tap the right hand with my finger, to encourage it to rise. Don't give up unless the client gives up. If you have zero success, you have a client who has some blockage. In this case, ask them to relax, and invite them to describe the most peaceful scene they can imagine, for about 3 minutes, then continue to step 9. Most clients will raise the hand, and I will congratulate them, and even clap my hands, saying, *"Wonderful! This means your subconscious mind is going to help you quit smoking, by removing the cravings, and making it so easy to quit. When I count to 3, your right arm will fall gently to your side, and you will drop into the deepest sleep you have felt in a long time. 1,2,3, your right arm is now resting at your side, and you feel more relaxed than you felt before."*)

What if smoking cigarettes just vanished from your mind, just like a puff of smoke? How would you feel about that?

Breathe deeply. Your breath is your life. Lung disease is horrible, right? Do you know anyone who suffered lung disease from smoking?

Heart attacks are horrible, right? Do you know any smokers who had a heart attack?

Let's be good to ourselves. I want you to love yourself more, and care for your precious breath. Notice the way you are breathing now, the rise and fall of your chest, the way the air passes through your nose. This is life, and smoking is death. Stay away from death.

Smoking promises to relieve stress, but only temporarily. Meditation is proven to reduce your stress permanently. Have you ever tried meditation? Just google Beginning Meditation, and watch the YouTube videos that will guide you as a beginner.

Meditation will help calm your mind. You will learn how to ignore distracting thoughts, like the junkie thought of smoking a cigarette. Can you make a commitment to yourself, to practice meditation for at least 5 minutes a day, for the next 3 weeks? Good! I promise you, your stress levels will drop, you will feel happier, lighter, and best of all you will stop smoking for good.

Imagine you are at work, and you feel stressed. What can you do to feel better? (Suggest that the client do a mini-meditation, or a wakeful "nap". She can also listen to a peaceful song, or drink a cup of herbal tea.)

If you screw up and smoke a cigarette, what will you do? (Suggest that she simply pretend that it never happened, and continue seeing herself as a non-smoker. Nothing has changed except her Quit Day. She still has all the same reasons to quit as before. She cannot fail if she doesn't give up.)

If someone offers you a cigarette, what will you tell them? (She should smile and say, "No thanks, I quit.")

If you see someone smoking, how will that make you feel? (She should feel sad for them, because they are still trapped in the prison of nicotine addiction, and she is free.)

I want you to imagine that it's 5 years into the future. You have been a non-smoker for 5 years!
How do you feel?
What is different about your life now?
What advice do you have, for someone who wants to quit smoking?
What are some dreams and goals, that were put on hold, because of cigarettes, but now are possible, because you are a non-smoker?

We need to replace your bad habit with a good one. Some people substitute hard candy for cigarettes, or chewing gum, or breath mints. You can even have a piece of fruit instead of a cigarette. What will you choose as a substitute for smoking?

This is your new substitute, and you will have lots of hard candy (or gum) on hand and easy to reach. Whenever you feel an urge to smoke, just pop some delicious hard candy in your mouth, and you will feel more satisfied than when you smoked. The reason you will feel

MORE satisfied, is because you will feel the pride of successfully quitting cigarettes. You will feel your health improving, along with your confidence and self esteem. Those happy feelings are a thousand times better than a cigarette.

In what ways has smoking caused you pain?

I want you to imagine your favorite brand of cigarettes. Notice the design on the pack, and the stamp on the cigarette. Can you see it? Good.

I want you to see yourself putting a cigarette up to your lips, and lighting it. Now imagine the most disgusting taste has entered your mouth. The more gross it is, the better. Imagine the smell of raw sewage, and the taste of rotten food, this is what cigarettes will taste like for you, from now on.

The cigarette is so disgusting to you, it smells like a dead body. And cigarettes cause millions of deaths every year. You are so disgusted, you pull it from your mouth, and it leaves a black stain of poison on your lips! You are sickened by the whole experience, and you want nothing to do with smoking ever again.

You are a permanent nonsmoker now. You feel happy and satisfied, breathing clean, pure air.

You feel no cravings at all for cigarettes. Any discomfort you feel, is NOT your body asking for nicotine. The discomfort is your body HEALING itself, healing the damage done by years of smoking. When you feel this healing in your body, you will feel wonderful, because your body is becoming stronger, cleaner, and healthy.

When you see cigarettes at the store, you will feel lucky, that you are free from that dangerous addiction. When you see cigarette butts on the sidewalk, you will know that the person who tossed that butt is still trapped in a prison of tobacco. You have escaped, and you feel free and wonderful.

When you see someone smoking, you will feel sorry for them. They don't smoke of their own free will. They are slaves to tobacco, and you are lucky to be free of that pain.

You know, in your heart of hearts, that smoking is destructive, dangerous, and unhealthy. Unhealthy thoughts have no place in your life, or your mind. Ignore any unhealthy thought...ignore everything about smoking and I promise you, those thoughts will get weaker and *weaker, until they disappear completely.*

I want you to imagine yourself, as a little girl, the way you used to look, when you were just 7 years old. (If client is a man, imagine a little boy) Remember the way you used to wear your hair, when you were 7, the style of clothes you wore, and the way you smiled back then. Can you see this little girl in your mind? Good. Please describe her to me. Tell me about her friends, her favorite games and toys, and her favorite memories.

Do you love this little girl? (90% will say yes. If client says NO, find out why. Usually she was abused and feels guilt or shame. If so, you must explore those feelings, bring them to the surface, and ask her to forgive the abuser, and herself, for everything. Only then can you proceed. This may take more than 1 session.)

This little girl needs your help. She is unhappy, because smoking is making her unhealthy. Your smoking is killing her. She doesn't want to die.

Do you love her enough to save her life? Good!

Imagine that you are standing in front of this beautiful little girl, who loves you deeply. See yourself telling her that you love her. Tell her that you will protect her from the dangers of smoking. Tell her she doesn't have to be afraid of cancer and heart attacks anymore.

Ask this beautiful little girl, if she will help you quit smoking, by making the cravings disappear, and making it easy to ignore thoughts of smoking. Now wait for her to reply, and when she does please share her answer with me. (The answer will be YES)

Wonderful! This little girl is going to help you quit. I want you to see yourself walking up to this little girl, and giving her a hug. Can you see her in your arms? Good. Hug her real close, so she feels the love you have for her. You are taller than she is, see yourself kissing the top of her head. Beautiful. Now hug her tighter, closer, so close that the two of you become one person.

Keep your promise to this little girl, she lives in your heart now, and she will help you so you never want to smoke again.

In a moment I will emerge you from hypnosis. When I count to 5 you will be wide awake, eyes open, feeling great. Most importantly, you will never want a disgusting cigarette again, and you won't think about smoking at all. 1,2,3,4,5, eyes open, wide awake, feeling great.

Weight Loss Script

(You have just spent days reading my book about hypnosis. Now you can use this script to hypnotize someone who wants to lose weight. Words in regular print are instructions, words in italics are spoken to the client. You should pepper your hypnosis session with LOTS of suggestions from my chapter in this book, "Patter". I want you to succeed, so if you have any questions at all, just email me and I will help you. FunWithHypnosis@gmail.com)

1. Ask Client to take a deep breathe, and close her eyes.

2. (Arm Heaviness Convincer) Ask her to raise her right arm straight up above her head, with her right fist closed tightly. *I want you to imagine you are holding a heavy bag, filled with sand. This bag is a brown canvas bag, and it's full of sand. This bag weighs over 10 pounds. Imagine what it feels like, to hold this heavy bag filled with sand high above your head. Can you see this bag in your mind's eye? Good. Imagine the weight of this bag of sand, pulling down on your arm as you strain to hold it. Can you feel the tension in the muscles of your shoulder, arm, and in the tiny muscles of your hand and fingers? Good, you are doing perfectly. When I count to 3 your arm will drop safely to your side, and you will enter a deep sleep. 1,2,3, your arm is now safely at your side, and you feel a deep relaxation.*

3. (Eye Lock Convincer) *I want you to focus your attention on the tiny muscles around your eyes. Focus all your attention on*

your eyelids, and give them permission to relax completely. It helps if you imagine that your eyelids are also heavy bags filled with sand. Allow your eyelids to relax so much, that they will not open. And when you are sure you've relaxed them so much, that they will not open, go ahead and give them a little test, and you will see that they will not open. (Wait for 2 seconds) Good, you can stop trying and keep your eyelids closed, and let yourself relax completely.

4. Let this relaxing feeling in your eyelids spread to the other muscles in your face, softening your expression, gently releasing any pockets of tension, in your neck and throat. Your shoulders are dropping now, slipping into a sleepy posture, and your arms are loose, limp, and relaxed, so comfortable and sleepy.

5. Your breathing is slow and regular, like the breathing of a sleeping person. Hypnosis is just like sleep, except you will always be able to hear my voice, and respond to my words. Your heart is beating softer, and a heavy sleepy feeling is spreading to every part of your body.

6. (Fractionation) In a moment I will ask you to open your eyes, and find a spot on the ceiling to stare at. You can choose any spot that suits you. Then I will ask you to close your eyes. Are you ready? OK, open your eyes and find a spot on the ceiling to stare at. Focus all your attention on that spot, ignoring any other distractions, blocking out all sensations. Now close your eyes, and feel yourself drifting deeper into sleepy relaxation. (Do this 3 times)

7. (Look at your client. If she seems deeply relaxed, skip step 8)

8. (Losing the Numbers) *In a moment I'm going to ask you to count backward from 100. But you will count in a special way. You will count like this, "100, deeper sleep, 99, deeper sleep, 98, deeper sleep," and so on. But these numbers are special, because very soon they will drop out of your mind, fade away, and disappear. When that happens, just stop counting, and relax. Are you ready to begin? Good. Start counting backwards for me now.* (Every number she counts, you say things like, "Slower...Softer....Sleep is coming....The numbers are fading....The numbers are gone...." When she makes a long pause, or stops completely, say, "The numbers have dropped from your mind, you can stop counting and relax.")

9. (Arm Float Convincer) *I am speaking to your subconscious mind now, to your inner mind. As you think about your desire to lose weight easily, your right arm is going to start to rise, float, levitate straight up towards the ceiling. The more intensely you desire freedom from poor health and overeating, the faster your right arm will rise, the higher it will rise. Don't assist it and don't resist it, just let it happen naturally, as you focus all your attention on breaking free from the pain of being overweight. Imagine all the wonderful things you can do, without health problems of any kind to slow you down. And as your right arm rises higher and higher, your inner mind is declaring the same desire, for an end to the shame of over-eating, and its emotional pain.* (Keep suggesting the phrases in this step, until the arm rises high. I like to tap the right hand with my finger, to encourage it to rise. Don't give up unless the client gives up. If you have zero success, you have a client who has some blockage. In this case, ask them to relax, and invite them to describe the most peaceful scene they can imagine, for about 3 minutes, then continue to step 9. Most clients will raise the hand, and I will congratulate them, and even clap my hands, saying, *"Wonderful! This means your subconscious mind is going to help you lose the weight, by removing the cravings for sugary snacks and fatty foods, and making it so easy to drop the weight. When I count to 3, your right arm will fall gently to your side, and you will drop into the deepest sleep you have felt in a long time. 1,2,3, your right arm is now resting at your side, and you feel more relaxed than you felt before."*)

How long have you been struggling with your weight?
What are some ways that being overweight has caused you to feel unhealthy or unhappy?

As you think back in your life, what is the one accomplishment that you feel most proud of? Something that was difficult to achieve, something you feel so proud of? Remember this feeling, because this is what you are going to feel, when you lose all the weight you want. Tell me how that will make you feel, when you step on the scale, and you have lost 40 pounds.

I want you to imagine your favorite sugary snack. What is it? (Let's pretend she says "Cake.") *Notice the design on the box of cake, and really see this cake in your mind. Can you see it? Good.*

I want you to see yourself putting a fork into the cake, and bringing a bite up to your lips, and putting it in your mouth. Now imagine the most disgusting taste has entered your mouth. The more gross it is, the better. Imagine the smell of raw sewage, and the taste of rotten food, this is what sugary and fattening foods will taste like for you, from now on.

Sugary food is so disgusting to you, it smells like a dead body. And fattening foods cause millions of deaths every year. You are so disgusted, you can't swallow it, so you spit it out, and it leaves a black stain of poison on your lips! You are sickened by the whole experience, and you want nothing to do with fattening foods ever again.

From this very moment, starting right now, you no longer have the urge to overeat, or to snack in between meals. Healthy, well balanced meals satisfy you completely. Rich, heavy, sweet, fattening foods just no longer appeal to you, in fact they make you nauseous.

From now on, you chew your food noticeably slower, savoring every bite, taking your time, so you eat much less, but enjoy your food more.

You can snack all you want, on fresh fruit. There is no reason for you to feel hungry, because you can eat all the fresh fruit you want. What are your favorite fresh fruits?

You will eat 3 sensible meals a day, and all the fresh fruit you like. If you still feel hungry, that is your Overeating Voice talking. You need to ignore this voice, and I promise you it will get weaker and weaker until it disappears.

I want you to imagine that it's 1 year into the future. You have lost 40 pounds! This is a total victory over your weight loss goals. What does that feel like? How will your life change, when you lose this weight?

I want you to imagine yourself, as a little girl, the way you used to look, when you were just 7 years old. (If client is a man, imagine a little boy) *Remember the way you used to wear your hair, when you were 7, the style of clothes you wore, and the way you smiled back then. Can you see this little girl in your mind? Good. Please describe her to me. Tell me about her friends, her favorite games and toys, and her favorite memories.*

Do you love this little girl? (90% will say yes. If client says NO, find out why. Usually she was abused and feels guilt or shame. If so, you must explore those feelings, bring them to the surface, and ask her to forgive the abuser, and herself, for everything. Only then can you proceed. This may take more than 1 session.)

This little girl needs your help. She is unhappy, because overeating is making her unhealthy. Your emotional eating is making her feel sad. She doesn't want to be overweight.

Do you love her enough to save her life? Good!

Imagine that you are standing in front of this beautiful little girl, who loves you deeply. See yourself telling her that you love her. Tell her that you will protect her from the dangers of a poor diet. Tell her she doesn't have to be afraid of poor health.

Ask this beautiful little girl, if she will help you lose weight, by making the cravings for bad snacks disappear, and making it easy for you to exercise. Now wait for her to reply, and when she does please share her answer with me. (The answer will be YES)

Wonderful! This little girl is going to help you diet. I want you to see yourself walking up to this little girl, and giving her a hug. Can you see her in your arms? Good. Hug her real close, so she feels the love you have for her. You are taller than she is, see yourself kissing the top of her head. Beautiful. Now hug her tighter, closer, so close that the two of you become one person.

Keep your promise to this little girl, she lives in your heart now, and she will help you so you lose all the weight you want, and feel healthy and fit and trim.

In a moment I will emerge you from hypnosis. When I count to 5 you will be wide awake, eyes open, feeling great. Most importantly, you will never want a disgusting cigarette again, and you won't think about smoking at all. 1,2,3,4,5, eyes open, wide awake, feeling great.

Thank you for reading my book!

I would love to hypnotize you, for any positive purpose. If you are on a budget, I can reduce of waive the fee. I just want to help you live a better life.

If you are interested in learning how to hypnotize people, I am happy to help you and share my knowledge and experience. No charge.

Thanks Again,

Alex the Hypnotist

FunWithHypnosis@gmail.com